Echocardiography in Diseases

Echocardiography in Diseases

Edited by **Mckinsey Harper**

hayle
medical

New York

Published by Hayle Medical,
30 West, 37th Street, Suite 612,
New York, NY 10018, USA
www.haylemedical.com

Echocardiography in Diseases
Edited by Mckinsey Harper

International Standard Book Number: 978-1-63241-113-6 (Hardback)

Contents

Permissions

List of Contributors

Preface

Over the recent decade, advancements and applications have progressed exponentially. This has led to the increased interest in this field and projects are being conducted to enhance knowledge. The main objective of this book is to present some of the critical challenges and provide insights into possible solutions. This book will answer the varied questions that arise in the field and also provide an increased scope for furthering studies.

The book offers an in-depth look at echocardiography, elucidating its role in diseases. It is a compilation of research works by international researchers; some of them specializing in imaging science in their clinical orientation, and others, representatives from academic medical centers. The book has been structured and written with such simplicity that it will be understandable to readers with basic knowledge of echocardiography and will also be stimulating and informative to experts and researchers in the field of echocardiography. This book targets readers involved in cardiology during their basic echocardiography rotation, internal medicine, radiology and emergency medicine and also to specialists in echocardiography. During the past few decades, technological advancements in echocardiography have evolved rapidly, leading to improved echocardiographic imaging using new techniques. The role of echocardiography in several special pathologies has also been discussed by several authors in the book.

I hope that this book, with its visionary approach, will be a valuable addition and will promote interest among readers. Each of the authors has provided their extraordinary competence in their specific fields by providing different perspectives as they come from diverse nations and regions. I thank them for their contributions.

Editor

Part 1

Echocardiography in Valvular Heart Disease

Echocardiography in Severe Aortic Stenosis

Gani Bajraktari
Service of Cardiology, University Clinical Centre of Kosova, Prishtina
Republic of Kosovo

1. Introduction

Aortic stenosis (AS) is the most frequent valvular heart disease in west developed and developing countries, with prevalence between 0.02% in adults under 44 years and 3-9% in elderly over 80 years. Patients with this disease may remain asymptomatic for years, particularly in elderly with naturally limited exercise. If the patients remain untreated after they become symptomatic, the mortality at 10 years follow-up is 80-90%. Based on the etiology, mainly are three types of AS: 1) Calcific AS, which is most frequent type in adults of advanced age (2–7% of the population), 2) Congenital, which dominates in the younger patients, and 3) Rheumatic AS, which is becoming rare in developed countries.

Patient history and physical examination remain important in the diagnosis of AS. For the proper patient management, the evidence of the symptoms characteristic for AS: exertional shortness of breath, angina, dizziness, or syncope. Further diagnostic right direction is characteristic systolic murmur.

The disappearance of the second aortic sound is specific to severe AS.

Aortic valve replacement (AVR) is the only effective treatment for severe aortic AS. It is performed either isolated or concomitantly with coronary artery by-pass graft operation, which take place in almost 50% of patients with AS. The overall mortality of isolated AVR is 3-5% in patients below 70 years and 5-15% in elderly. After successful AVR, symptoms and quality of live improves significantly. The long term 10 years survival after successful AVR is very satisfied and it resulted till 75%. The most important factors that may affect the survival are old age, high NYHA functional class, associated aortic regurgitation, concomitant coronary aortic by-pass graft and atrial fibrillation.

2. Echocardiography in aortic stenosis patients

Echocardiography is the key diagnostic tool, not only to confirm the presence of AS, but also to assesses the degree of valve calcification, LV function and wall thickness. Today, echocardiography provides prognostic information in patients with AS.

The severity of AS is provided with a very high sensitivity and specificity by Doppler echocardiography. A valve area 1.0 cm^2 in a patient with AS is considered severe. The indexing of aortic valve area to body surface area is more powerful parameter, and a cut-off value of 0.6 cm^2/m^2 is considered severe AS. However, valve area detected by Doppler echocardiography cannot be the only parameter for clinical decision making for aortic valve replacement, and it should be considered in combination with flow rate, pressure gradient and ventricular function, as well as functional status of an individual patient.

In patients with AS and normal left ventricular (LV) ejection fraction (EF) the mean pressure gradient of 50 mmHg (Figure 1), was used as a cut-off for the decision making for aortic valve replacement. However, in patients with depressed global LV function, even in patients with severe AS, Doppler echocardiography may result with low pressure gradients (underestimated gradients). In these patients, stress echocardiography using low-dose dobutamine may be helpful to distinguish truly severe AS patients from the rare cases of pseudosevere AS. In patients with truly severe AS, only small changes in valve area, but significant increase in pressure gradients are shown, whereas in pseudosevere AS patients are registered significant increase of valve area surface, but only minor changes in pressure gradients, before and at peak dose of dobutamine. The dobutamine stress-echocardiography is useful also to detect the presence of contractile reserve, which has prognostic implications.

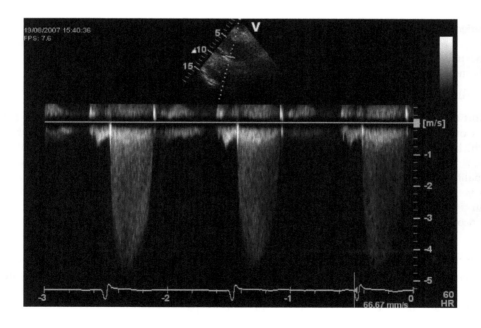

Fig. 1. Continues Doppler velocity of the aortic valve, in a patient with high pressure gradient and normal EF, before aortic valve replacement.

3. Outcome of patients with aortic stenosis

Aortic stenosis is a chronic progressive disease. Patients with AS may remain asymptomatic for a long period of time, and the duration of the asymptomatic phase varies widely among individuals. The most frequent cause of death in symptomatic patients is sudden cardiac death. However, sudden cardiac death in asymptomatic patients with AS is very rare.

Older age, presence of atherosclerotic risk factors, valve calcification, peak aortic jet velocity, low LV EF and increase of transvalvular pressure gradient with exercise, were shown as independent predictors of poor outcome in AS patients.

The development of symptoms on exercise testing, in physically active patients with AS, predicts a very high likelihood of symptom development within 12 months. The occurrence of symptoms, in these patientsş is a correlate of poor prognosis. The increased of mortality in these patients has been reported within months of symptom onset, which is often not promptly reported by patients.

4. Echocardiographic predictors in patients with severe aortic stenosis and poor left ventricular systolic function

Left ventricular systolic function was shown as one of more important predictors of patients with AS. Patients with AS and LV systolic dysfunction have a poor prognosis if valve replacement is not performed. LV EF, as the most important conventional parameter for the LV global systolic function, was consistently reported as a postoperative prognostic factor in patients with severe AS. Patients with severe left ventricular dysfunction have increased intra-operative mortality, and there are yet contradictions about their improved outcomes after the AVR. Generally, the LV systolic dysfunction is not a contraindication to surgery. It was shown that patients who underwent AVR have a 5-year survival rate 60–70%, with a high operative mortality in the range of 10–15% for patients with LV systolic dysfunction. To predict the postoperative outcome of patients with severe AS and impaired LV function, the preoperative dobutamine stress echocardiography is useful technique. The presence of good contractile reserve in dobutamine stress echocardiography supports potential benefit from AVR and better outcome in these patients.

AVR decreases the LV afterload, through transvalvular pressure drop (Figure 2), resulting in regression of LV hypertrophy.

LV mass regression predominantly occurs within the first 6 months of surgery. Even there are few publications regarding the pre-operative echocardiographic predictors of LV functional recovery in AS patients with low EF, it justify the statement to consider these patients for the operation, after individual assessment of the patient, considering co morbidities and general conditions.

Recovery of LV function was evident after aortic valve replacement in the majority of patients with aortic stenosis and pre-operative LV dysfunction.

Patients with increased LV end-systolic dimension and/or LV systolic volume index seem to have less chance for the LV functional recovery. It seems that these patients loosed contractile reserve, and up to now there is no evidence that they may improve LV systolic function after operation, and therefore we should less encourage these patients for the AVR. However, there are studies that have shown that even in patients with poor LV systolic function, there is still ability for a LV function recovery after AVR, explaining it through the mechanism of the markedly reduction of outflow tract resistance.

Studies have shown that stented and stentless valves have similar effect on the LV mass reduction after AVR in all patients that underwent this procedure, despite significant differences in indexed effective orifice area and peak flow velocity in favor of the stentless valve. However, in patients with AS and markedly reduced ventricular function, there was shown more rapid LV mass and function normalization in stentless patients compared to similar patients receiving a stented valve. The luck of large randomized studies for these prostheses makes even more difficult decision. However, a numerous retrospective studies have shown improvement in symptoms and LV EF in about 70% of the survivors after AVR in patients with low LV EF.

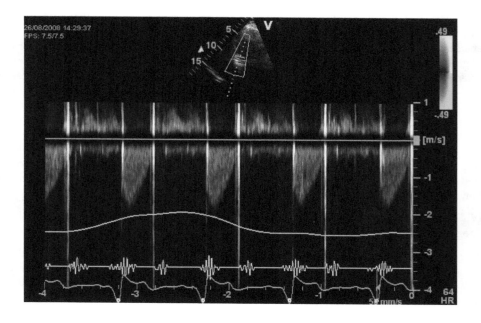

Fig. 2. Continues Doppler velocity of the aortic valve, in the same patient, two weeks after aortic valve replacement.

They suggest that despite increased operative mortality, these patients should not be denied aortic valve replacement, given the substantial potential clinical benefit from AVR replacement.

In conclusion, in patients with severe aortic stenosis with impaired LV global systolic function, assessed by LV EF, AVR has significantly better outcome compared to those treated medically. These patients are likely to carry a high risk operation (up to 10%), than to have a very poor prognosis for 10 years survival in medical treatment.

5. Echocardiographic predictors in patients with severe aortic stenosis and preserved left ventricular systolic function

Global LV function, assessed by conventional EF remains normal in most of AS patients. However, the long axis systolic function, assessed by M-mode echocardiography and/or tissue Doppler imaging (TDI) velocities, decreases even in patients with preserved EF. In AS patients with preserved EF, the longitudinal velocity, strain and strain rate are decreased and deteriorate further as AS become severe. These changes reflect that the LV myocardial dysfunction beginning at the subendocardium in early stages of AS and progress to mid-wall and to transmural contraction impairment in patients with severe AS. Recent studies have shown also that in patients with AS and preserved LV EF, the apical rotation and LV twist are increased and untwist is delayed compared to normals, as compensatory mechanisms for the increased intracavitary pressure overload and subendocardial ischaemia. Also, it was shown that these LV myocardial correlate with the severity of AS. However, these compensatory mechanisms are lost after the LV EF deterioration.

Strong evidence exists showing beneficial effect of AVR, not only in improving patients' symptoms but also in recovering, even partially, overall cardiac function. Improvement of LV ventricular function in these patients is interpreted on the basis of regression of myocardial hypertrophy, increased myocardial perfusion and hence overall cavity performance, at early and mid-term post-operative periods. While EF is the most popular measure of pre-operative LV systolic function in such patients, and surgical risk assessment it lacks representing subendocardial component of the LV function.

Severe aortic stenosis causes significant subendocardial dysfunction despite preserved ejection fraction. Aortic valve replacement surgery and removal of left ventricular afterload results in recovery of intrinsic subendocardial function within a week of surgery, well before mass regression and reverse remodeling. Such degree of pre-operative subendocardial disturbances may represent early changes that if ignored may substantiate and become irreversible. Thus, the presence of such abnormalities in symptomatic patients, even with normal ejection fraction, may suggest further evidence for a need for valve replacement in order to maintain overall integral ventricular function and to avoid potential clinical complications.

In patients with severe aortic stenosis and and maintained LV EF, the left ventricular twist is increased as compared with normal subjects suggesting a wall motion compensation for the reduced long axis motion in the aim to preserve LVEF. These motions alter towards normal values within six months of aortic valve replacement (Figure 3). These findings are growing evidence that on LV dysfunction and their improvement after AVR, even in asymptomatic patients, and may assist in identifying patients needing surgery before LV damage becomes irreversible.

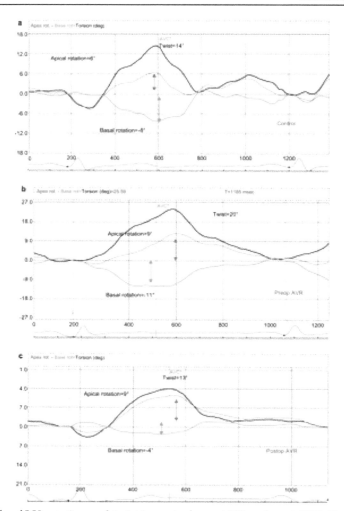

Fig. 3. Example of LV rotation and twist in control, pre AVR and post AVR. Purple line showing peak of apical rotation and green showing peak basal rotation. AVR, aortic valve replacement (Reproduced from *Lindqvist P et al.* Aortic valve replacement normalizes left ventricular twist function. Interact CardioVasc Thorac Surg 2011;12:701-706, doi:10.1510/icvts.2010.262303, with permission from the European Association for Cardio-Thoracic Surgery).

6. References

[1] Iung B, Baron G, Butchart EG, Delahaye F, Gohlke-Barwolf C, Levang OW, Tornos P, Vanoverschelde JL, Vermeer F, Boersma E, Ravaud P, Vahanian A. A prospective survey of patients with valvular heart disease in Europe: the Euro Heart Survey on valvular heart disease. Eur Heart J 2003; 24: 1231-1243.

[2] Stewart BF, Siscovick D, Lind BK, Gardin JM, Gottdiener JS, Smith VE, Kitzman DW, Otto CM. Clinical factors associated with calcific aortic valve disease. Cardiovascular Health Study. J Am Coll Cardiol 1997; 29: 630–634.

[3] Vahanian A, Baumgartner H, Bax J, Butchart E, Dion R, Filippatos G, Flachskampf F, Hall R, Iung B, Kasprzak J, Nataf P, Tornos P, Torracca L, Wenink A; Task Force on the Management of Valvular Hearth Disease of the European Society of Cardiology; ESC Committee for Practice Guidelines. Guidelines on the management of valvular heart disease: The Task Force on the Management of Valvular Heart Disease of the European Society of Cardiology. Eur Heart J 2007; 28: 230-68.

[4] Quinones MA, Otto CM, Stoddard M, Waggoner A, Zoghbi WA, for the Doppler Quantification Task Force of the Nomenclature Standards Committee of the American Society of Echocardiography. Recommendations for quantification of Doppler echocardiography: a report from the Doppler Quantification Task Force of the Nomenclature and Standards Committee of the American Society of Echocardiography. J Am Soc Echocardiogr 2002; 15: 167-184.

[5] deFilippi CR, Willett DL, Brickner ME, Appleton CP, Yancy CW, Eichhorn EJ, Grayburn PA. Usefulness of dobutamine echocardiography in distinguishing severe from nonsevere valvular aortic stenosis in patients with depressed left ventricular function and low transvalvular gradients. Am J Cardiol 1995; 75: 191-194.

[6] Nishimura RA, Grantham JA, Connolly HM, Schaff HV, Higano ST, Holmes DR Jr. Low-output, low-gradient aortic stenosis in patients with depressed left ventricular systolic function: the clinical utility of the dobutamine challenge in the catheterization laboratory. Circulation 2002; 106: 809-813.

[7] Monin JL, Quere JP, Monchi M, Petit H, Baleynaud S, Chauvel C, Pop C, Ohlmann P, Lelguen C, Dehant P, Tribouilloy C, Gueret P. Low-gradient aortic stenosis, operative risk stratification and predictors for long-term outcome: a multicenter study using dobutamine stress hemodynamics. Circulation 2003; 108:319-324.

[8] Rosenhek R, Binder T, Porenta G, Lang I, Christ G, Schemper M, Maurer G, Baumgartner H. Predictors of outcome in severe, asymptomatic aortic stenosis. N Engl J Med 2000; 343: 611-617.

[9] Pellikka PA, Sarano ME, Nishimura RA, Malouf JF, Bailey KR, Scott CG, Barnes ME, Tajik AJ. Outcome of 622 adults with asymptomatic, hemodynamically significant aortic stenosis during prolonged follow-up. Circulation 2005; 111: 3290-3295.

[10] Amato MC, Moffa PJ, Werner KE, Ramires JA. Treatment decision in asymptomatic aortic valve stenosis: role of exercise testing. Heart 2001; 86: 381-386.

[11] Bruch C, Stypmann J, Grude M, Gradaus R, Breithardt G, Wichter T. Tissue Doppler imaging in patients with moderate to severe aortic valve stenosis: clinical usefulness and diagnostic accuracy. Am Heart J 2004; 148: 696-702.

[12] Tarantini G, Buja P, Scognamiglio R, Razzolini R, Gerosa G, Isabella G, Ramondo A, Iliceto S. Aortic valve replacement in severe aortic stenosis with left ventricular dysfunction: determinants of cardiac mortality and ventricular function recovery. Eur J Cardiothorac Surg 2003; 24: 879-85.

[13] Kupari M, Turto H, Lommi J. Left ventricular hypertrophy in aortic valve stenosis: preventive or promotive of systolic dysfunction and heart failure? Eur Heart J 2005; 26: 1790-6.

[14] Das P, Rimington H, Chambers J. Exercise testing to stratify risk in aortic stenosis. Eur Heart J 2005; 26: 1309-1313.

[15] Lancellotti P, Lebois F, Simon M, Tombeux C, Chauvel C, Pierard LA. Prognostic importance of quantitative exercise Doppler echocardiography in asymptomatic valvular aortic stenosis. Circulation 2005; 112(Suppl. I): I-377–I-382.

[16] Lund O, Nielsen TT, Emmertsen K, Flo C, Rasmussen B, Jensen FT, Pilegaard HK, Kristensen LH, Hansen OK. Mortality and worsening of prognostic profile during waiting time for valve replacement in aortic stenosis. Thorac Cardiovasc Surg 1996; 44: 289-295.

[17] Collinson J, Flather M, Coats AJ, Pepper JR, Henein M. Influence of valve prosthesis type on the recovery of ventricular dysfunction and subendocardial ischaemia following valve replacement for aortic stenosis. Int J Cardiol 2004; 97: 535-41.

[18] Arshad W, Duncan AM, Francis DP, O'Sullivan CA, Gibson DG, Henein MY. Opposite effects of coronary artery disease and hypertrophic cardiomyopathy on left ventricular long axis function during dobutamine stress. Int J Cardiol 2005; 101: 123-8.

[19] Pereira JJ, Lauer MS, Bashir M, Afridi I, Blackstone EH, Stewart WJ, McCarthy PM, Thomas JD, Asher CR. Survival after aortic valve replacement for severe aortic stenosis with low transvalvular gradients and severe left ventricular dysfunction. J Am Coll Cardiol 2002; 39: 1356-63.

[20] Takeda S, Rimington H, Smeeton N, Chambers J. Long axis excursion in aortic stenosis. Heart 2001; 86: 52-6.

[21] Blackstone EH, Cosgrove DM, Jamieson WR, Birkmeyer NJ, Lemmer JH Jr, Miller DC, Butchart EG, Rizzoli G, Yacoub M, Chai A. Prosthesis size and long-term survival after aortic valve replacement. J Thorac Cardiovasc Surg 2003; 126: 783-96.

[22] Carabello BA. Evaluation and management of patients with aortic stenosis. Circulation 2002; 105:1746–50.

[23] Vaquette B, Corbineau H, Laurent M, Lelong B, Langanay T, de Place C, Froger-Bompas C, Leclercq C, Daubert C, Leguerrier A. Valve replacement in patients with critical aortic stenosis and depressed left ventricular function: predictors of operative risk, left ventricular function recovery, and long term outcome. Heart 2005; 91: 1324-9.

[24] Perez de Arenaza D, Lees B, Flather M, Nugara F, Husebye T, Jasinski M, Cisowski M, Khan M, Henein M, Gaer J, Guvendik L, Bochenek A, Wos S, Lie M, Van Nooten G, Pennell D, Pepper J; ASSERT (Aortic Stentless versus Stented valve assessed by Echocardiography Randomized Trial) Investigators. Randomized comparison of stentless versus stented valves for aortic stenosis: effects on left ventricular mass. Circulation 2005; 112: 2696-702.

[25] Ding WH, Lam YY, Kaya MG, Li W, Chung R, Pepper JR, Henein MY. Echocardiographic predictors of left ventricular functional recovery following

valve replacement surgery for severe aortic stenosis. Int J Cardiol 2008; 128: 178-84.

[26] Lim E, Ali A, Theodorou P, Sousa I, Ashrafian H, Chamageorgakis T, Duncan A, Henein M, Diggle P, Pepper J. Longitudinal study of the profile and predictors of left ventricular mass regression after stentless aortic valve replacement. Ann Thorac Surg 2008; 85: 2026-9.

[27] Cramariuc D, Gerdts E, Davidsen ES, Segadal L, Matre K. Myocardial deformation in aortic valve stenosis: relation to left ventricular geometry. Heart 2010; 96: 106-12.

[28] Dinh W, Nickl W, Smettan J, Kramer F, Krahn T, Scheffold T, Barroso MC, Brinkmann H, Koehler T, Lankisch M, Füth R. Reduced global longitudinal strain in association to increased left ventricular mass in patients with aortic valve stenosis and normal ejection fraction: a hybrid study combining echocardiography and magnetic resonance imaging. Cardiovasc Ultrasound 2010; 8: 29.

[29] Ding WH, Lam YY, Pepper JR, Kaya MG, Li W, Chung R, Henein MY. Early and long-term survival after aortic valve replacement in septuagenarians and octogenarians with severe aortic stenosis. Int J Cardiol 2010; 141: 24-31.

[30] Ding WH, Lam YY, Duncan A, Li W, Lim E, Kaya MG, Chung R, Pepper JR, Henein MY. Predictors of survival after aortic valve replacement in patients with low-flow and high-gradient aortic stenosis. Eur J Heart Fail 2009; 11: 897-902.

[31] Lindqvist P, Bajraktari G, Molle R, Palmerini E, Holmgren A, Mondillo S, Henein MY. Valve replacement for aortic stenosis normalizes subendocardial function in patients with normal ejection fraction. Eur J Echocardiogr 2010; 11: 608-13

[32] Zhao Y, Lindqvist P, Nilsson J, Holmgren A, Näslund U, Henein MY. Trans-catheter aortic valve implantation--early recovery of left and preservation of right ventricular function. Interact Cardiovasc Thorac Surg 2011; 12: 35-9.

[33] Lindqvist P, Zhao Y, Bajraktari G, Holmgren A, Henein MY. Aortic valve replacement normalizes left ventricular twist function. Interact Cardiovasc Thorac Surg 2011; 12: 701-6.

[34] Owen A, Henein MY. Challenges in the management of severe asymptomatic aortic stenosis. Eur J Cardiothorac Surg 2011; 40: 848-50.

[35] Lam YY, Bajraktari G, Lindqvist P, Holmgren A, Mole R, Li W, Duncan A, Ding WH, Mondillo S, Pepper JR, Henein MY. Prolonged total isovolumic time is related to reduced long-axis functional recovery following valve replacement surgery for severe aortic stenosis. Int J Cardiol 2011. [Epub ahead of print]

[36] Zhao Y, Lindqvist P, Holmgren A, Henein MY. Accentuated left ventricular lateral wall function compensates for septal dyssynchrony after valve replacement for aortic stenosis. Int J Cardiol. 2011 Jul 30. [Epub ahead of print]

[37] Strain analysis in patients with severe aortic stenosis and preserved left ventricular ejection fraction undergoing surgical valve replacement. Delgado V, Tops LF, van Bommel RJ, van der Kley F, Marsan NA, Klautz RJ, Versteegh MI, Holman ER, Schalij MJ, Bax JJ. Eur Heart J 2009; 30: 3037-47.

[38] Miyazaki S, Daimon M, Miyazaki T, Onishi Y, Koiso Y, Nishizaki Y, Ichikawa R, Chiang SJ, Makinae H, Suzuki H, Daida H.Global longitudinal strain in relation to the severity of aortic stenosis: a two-dimensional speckle-tracking study. Echocardiography 2011; 28: 703-8.

[39] Ng AC, Delgado V, Bertini M, Antoni ML, van Bommel RJ, van Rijnsoever EP, van der Kley F, Ewe SH, Witkowski T, Auger D, Nucifora G, Schuijf JD, Poldermans D, Leung DY, Schalij MJ, Bax JJ. Alterations in multidirectional myocardial functions in patients with aortic stenosis and preserved ejection fraction: a two-dimensional speckle tracking analysis. Eur Heart J 2011; 32: 1542-50.

2

The Degenerative Mitral Valve Regurgitation: From Geometrical Echocardiographic Concepts to Successful Surgical Repair

Gheorghe Cerin, Bogdan Adrian Popa and Marco Diena
The Cardioteam Foundation / San Gaudenzio Clinic, Novara
Italy

1. Introduction

Echocardiography has become within the last years the main tool in the evaluation of the valvulopathies. Surgery plays a key role in the management of the valvular disorders, but it must be underlined that the surgical timing, planning and indication are all widely based on echocardiography. All the guidelines use the echocardiographic criteria to manage the valvular patients. Echocardiography became the main tool for the selection of the patient candidate to valve repair or replacement. The echocardiographic assessment is important in all the valvulopathies, but becomes crucial in the management of patients with mitral insufficiency, candidate to mitral valve repair.

Still, it should be noted, that there is no randomized study comparing the mitral valve repair and mitral valve replacement, and comparisons between the two, using propensity matching or other statistical methods are very difficult. On the other hand there are numerous studies which suggest that the short and long term outcomes of patients undergoing successful mitral valve repair are superior to those undergoing replacement.

Mitral valve repair has been proved to increase additional operative and long-term survival advantages over mitral valve replacement in case of chronic mitral regurgitation. The reduction in the left ventricular pump performance that has been observed after conventional mitral valve replacement, has not been obvious with mitral valve repair, provided that the postoperative contractile state remains pretty similar to the preoperative hemodynamic status. Compared to mitral replacement, mitral valve repair has lower mortality rates and higher long-term survival.. In addition, the thromboembolic and haemorrhagic complications associated with mitral valve reconstruction are also significantly decreased compared to mitral valve replacement. Several studies have reported that approximately 95% of patients are free from thromboembolic complications at 5 to 10 years after surgery. In contrast, 10% to 35% of patients with mechanical prostheses have thromboembolic events within 5 to 10 years after surgery (Bonow, 2011). Thus, the number of mitral valve repairs is expected to increase because the advantages over replacement were also clearly demonstrated by daily practice.

Nowadays, the number of patients undergoing mitral repair surgery is growing worldwide. The STS database proves that in the US, the percentage of patients undergoing mitral valve repair has increased from roughly 50% in 2000 to nearly 70% in 2007 (Bonow, 2011), for those patients with degenerative mitral regurgitation (excluding mitral stenosis, previous cardiac surgery and other types of surgery other than tricuspid valve procedures). The percentage of patients is expected to increase, considering that roughly 50% of the symptomatic patients with severe mitral regurgitation are still denied surgery. (Mirabel & colab,)

2. The role of echocardiography in the management of degenerative mitral regurgitation

First of all, in patients with degenerative mitral regurgitation, Echo identifies the type of degeneration: Barlow disease, fibroelastic deficiency (FED), hyper-elastic deficiency in Marfan syndrome etc. It is important for the surgeon to know it is important to know the aetiology of mitral insufficiency because some types of degenerative mitral regurgitation, such as FED, are more difficult to repair. Moreover, echo allows the identification of the mechanisms of mitral regurgitation, the alteration of leaflet coaptation and the specific geometrical concepts, which will be addressed further on.

In fact, echocardiography stands out as the only evaluation tool used in mitral valve repair. In dedicated centers, the tight collaboration between the echocardiographer and the surgeon, transformed the mitral valve repair into the gold standard treatment of mitral regurgitation, with over 90-95% of feasibility.

2.1 Standardization of the echocardiographic evaluation

The standardization of the perioperative echo exam is a key element; it allows the identification of specific patterns of lesions which consequently guide the surgical planning and determine the outcome. It may be considered that the standardisation of the echocardiographic lesions is, in fact, the first step to achieve a standardised surgical technique. At the very beginning, when the echocardiography was less powerful, the mitral repair and the surgical strategy were mainly done by direct anatomical assessment performed by the surgeon in the operating theatre, after opening of the left atrium. Over the last decade, due to to a better resolution of the echo machines and the experience of the echocardiographer, the method allowed a reliable assessment of mitral anatomy and lesions, and by doing so, permitted a reliable surgical planning before opening of the left atrium.

During the last decade, 'Cardioteam' has developed its own algorithm of mitral assessment, in order to standardize the lesions and the mechanisms of regurgitation. It uses some of the classically described patterns of lesions, such as mitral valve prolapse, flail, floppy or billowing mitral valve, but also new ones, such as 'undulating mitral valve', 'overturned' valve, 'marginal prolapse' of the anterior leaflet or 'pseudo-cleft' of the posterior leaflet. The application of this algorithm allowed a better understanding of the relationship between the mitral valve geometry and the valve function. This has significantly modified the surgical approach with subsequent improvement of the results.

Technically speaking, preoperative echocardiographic examination has to consider the mitral valve as an eight-component anatomical structure: three pairs of corresponding scallops (A_1-P_1, A_2-P_2, A_3-P_3) and the two commissures (Figure 1). This approach guarantees a better dialog with the surgical team, by mean of structured lesion localizations and standardization of the examination.

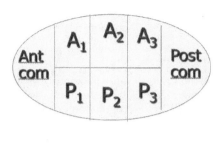

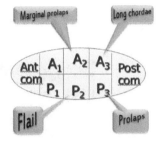

Fig. 1. The mitral valve scheme. The valve is divided into 8 components: three pairs of corresponding scallops (A_1-P_1, A_2-P_2, A_3-P_3) and two commissures. The Echo exam must describe the normality or the abnormalities of each component, assessing the pattern of mitral valve lesion for each one, focusing the attention on the leaflet coaptation.

2.2 The first step of standardization: The prolapsing score

During both transthoracic and intraoperative transesophageal examinations, each scallop must be analysed and a lesion code has to be ascribed: 0-normal, 1-elongated chordae, 2-prolapse, 3-flail and 4-marginal prolapse. The complexity of the valve disorders is expressed by the prolapsing score (PS), namely the ratio between the sick scallops and the total scallops (eg 1/8; 8/8) per patient (Cerin, 2006, 2010).

The echocardiographic message contained within the prolapsing score is fundamental for the surgeon to set the surgical approach. For example, when the echocardiographer states that the prolapsing score is 1/8 or 2/8, the surgical team expects a relatively 'simple' repair to be performed. Consequently, in such a patient the new surgical approaches such as minimally invasive surgery are more likely to be pursued. On the other hand, when the prolapsing score is as high as 8/8, the expected surgical approach will be different, more complex from the technical point of view, therefore more difficult and more likely to be done in classical sternotomy. In the operating theatre, the prolapsing score will be verified and confronted with the echo data Based on the experience of our center, around 75-80% of the echo information obtained from transthoracic exam fits the reality from the operating room.

2.3 The second step of standardization: Evaluation of the mitral valve geometry

The normal mitral geometry is the concept that guides both the evaluation of the various valve lesions and the surgical strategy. This is a key concept, also very helpful in the postoperative assessment of surgical result and for the echocardiographic follow up.

2.3.1 The triangle of coaptation

The central feature of the normal mitral valve geometry is represented by the triangle of coaptation (Cerin, 2006, Tesler 2009). It is usually assessed by two dimensional echocardiography and is delimited by the coaptation point, which is normally sited within the left ventricular cavity, and two other points placed on the septal and lateral mitral annulus (FIG 2). The triangle presents a height, which may be considered the expression of the optimal balance between the elastic and collagen fibres of the mitral valve. In patients with degenerative mitral valve, the height of the triangle of coaptation, which is usually reduced, expresses the excess of elastic fibres.

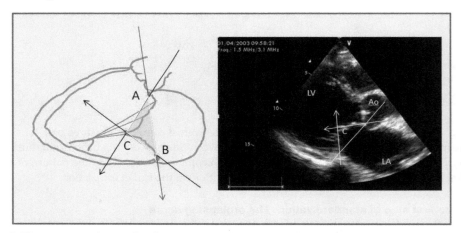

Fig. 2. The concept of triangle of coaptation. The triangle of coaptation is formed by the two points sited on the mitral annulus (A, B) and the coaptation point. The coaptation point (C) is normally situated into the left ventricle. LV – left ventricle; LA – left atrium; Ao – aorta;

At the tip of this triangle, the echocardiographer has to measure the length of leaflet coaptation. The coaptation length and the coaptation height are cornerstone elements used in order to fully describe the valve geometry and to assess the result of the repair.

It may be assumed that from a volumetric and a three dimensional geometrical perspective, the triangle of coaptation corresponds roughly to an asymmetrical tent. In the course of perioperative echocardiographic study, the systematic analysis of the mitral valve apparatus is done, focusing on whether the triangle of coaptation is present or not. The main surgical purpose of repair is achieving a good leaflet coaptation of at least 6mm in length and whenever possible, rebuilding the triangle of coaptation. Due to the increased amount of myxomatous tissue and elastic fibres in the mitral apparatus, the degenerative mitral valve usually loses its normal geometry progressively, alters the triangle of coaptation, presents itself as, elongated chordae or as a truly prolapsing valve.

2.4 The third step of standardization: Check the pattern of mitral valve lesions

In degenerative mitral insufficiency, many types of mitral valve lesions were classically described in the literature: from the classical mitral prolapse or mitral flail, to the billowing or floppy mitral valve. For a true dialogue between the echocardiographer, anaesthesiologist, and surgeon, all the team has to rigorously know the meaning of the most frequent lesions found in these patients. Alongside the well-known classically patterns of lesions, our group identifies some other particular patterns of mitral valve injuries, such as: elongated chordae, marginal prolapse, overturned mitral valve, undulating mitral valve or the mitral valve's pseudo-cleft. The main echocardiographic pattern used for the characterization of the degenerated mitral valve is presented further on.

2.4.1 The pattern of 'elongated chordae'

This pattern defines the situation when the coaptation point is found to be into the left ventricular cavity, immediately below the level of the mitral annulus. It is a borderline situation between a normal aspect of the mitral valve and the mitral prolapse. Usually is not associated with mitral regurgitation. For the surgical planning, it is important to recognise it and indicate it to the surgeon. Sometimes it may interest one or both leaflets (Figure 3), involving one or more scallops. The relatives of patients with truly mitral valve prolapse may sometimes present 'elongated chordae' during the echocardiographic exam, without the classical prolapse.

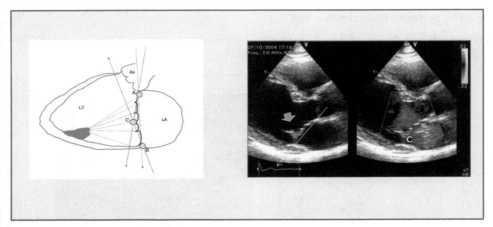

Fig. 3. The pattern of 'elongated chordae'. In the presence of 'elongated chordae', the coaptation point (C) is found into the left ventricular cavity, immediately below or at the level of the mitral annulus. Note the shape of the triangle of coaptation which is flattened. The coaptation height of the triangle has practically disappeared. LV – left ventricle; LA – left atrium; Ao – aorta.

2.4.2 The pattern of 'prolapsing valve'

The pattern of 'prolapsing valve' was classically defined as the presence of the coaptation point into the left atrium, above the level of the mitral annulus (Figure 4). By definition, the lesion has to be present in PSLAx view, otherwise, due to the shaded shape of the mitral valve, a false diagnose of mitral prolapse may be possible.

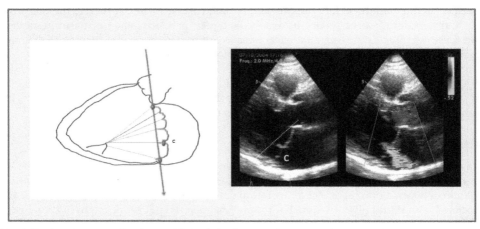

Fig. 4. Prolapsing mitral valve, with both leaflet involvement, shown in the 2D transthoracic parasternal long axis view. Notice the coaptation point (C) sited into the left atrium, behind the virtual line of the mitral annulus.

2.4.3 The pattern of mitral valve flail

It represents the classically loss of leaflet coaptation due to ruptured tendineous chordae. (Figure 5).

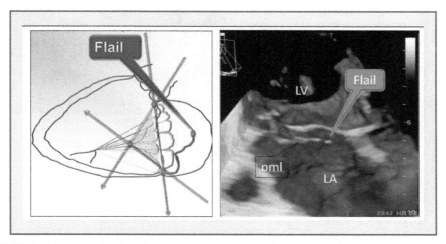

Fig. 5. Flail of the mitral valve shown in the transthoracic parasternal long axis view using real time three-dimensional technique (zoom). The classical lesion usually involves the P$_2$ scallop of the posterior leaflet, in about 2/3 of the patients with flail mitral valve. LA = left atrium, LV = left ventricle, pml = posterior mitral leaflet.

2.4.4 The pattern of 'marginal prolapse'

The pattern of 'marginal prolapse' is a rare type of mitral lesion, defined as an isolated protrusion of the free border area of one scallop, usually up to the insertion of the second degree chordae. In case of marginal prolapse, the remaining part of the surface of the scallop may be normal, without the displacement of the coaptation point into the left atrium. It is never present as isolated lesion; the marginal prolapse, as a rule, is associated with a P_2 scallop prolapse of the posterior leaflet (Figure 6).

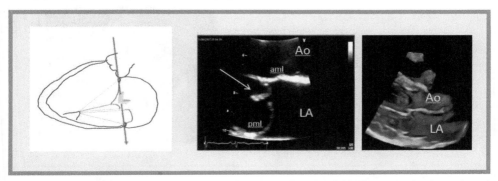

Fig. 6. Marginal prolapse of the anterior leaflet, A_2 scallop (arrow), shown in 2D (zoom) and 3 D Echo. Notice the "stair like aspect" of the anterior leaflet due to the regional prolapse located between the border of the valve and insertion of the second degree chordae (usually strut chordae). This is a hidden and tricky lesion, because its presence may transform the simple mitral plasty of one leaflet, in a complex mitral repair of both leaflets.

2.4.5 The 'undulating mitral valve'

The 'undulating mitral valve' is usually a redundant mitral valve, with excessive tissue, presenting with diastolic fluttering of the free border of both leaflets. In most cases, the prolapsing score is high, approximately 8/8 and as a rule, for the surgeon, it means a complex mitral repair. It is important to underline that the border or a normal mitral valve opens in a linear manner, without diastolic fluttering of the edge.

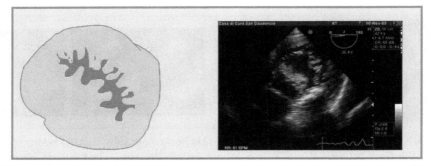

Fig. 7. Undulating mitral valve. TEE deep trans-gastric short axis view. Notice the undulating aspect of the free borders of the leaflets (much more evident on moving pictures).

2.4.6 The pattern of 'overturned mitral valve'

The pattern of 'overturned mitral valve': this kind of mitral lesion resembles the mitral valve flail as general echocardiographic aspect, but in the 'overturned mitral valve' the chordae are not ruptured (Figure 8). There is only an excessive elongation of the chordae and an obvious prolapse of the mitral valve into the left atrium.

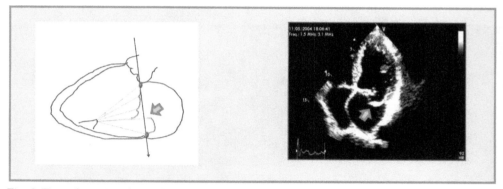

Fig. 8. Transthoracic echocardiography 4 chamber view, showing the obvious prolapse of the posterior mitral leaflet, due to the 'eversion' of the mitral valve. There is a loss of leaflet coaptation due to an excessive elongation of the mitral chordae (verified in the operating theatre).

2.4.7 The 'pseudo-cleft' of mitral valve

The 'pseudo-cleft' of mitral valve an obvious indentation of the border of the mitral valve, which penetrates deeply into the body of the mitral leaflet. It is pretty difficult to diagnose being visible only during the diastole and has to be integrated with the analyses of the colour Doppler in systole (Figure 9 A,B,C). It is never present as an isolated lesion; it is usually found in old mitral valve P_2 prolapse. A split which resembles a pseudo-cleft develops between the scallops P_2 and P_3 (or P_1).

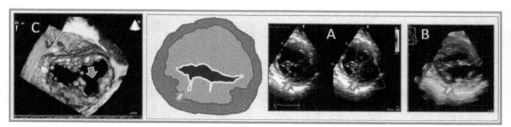

Fig. 9. (A,B,C). Diastolic transthoracic 2D and 3 D echocardiography short axis view (9A,B), showing the crack between P_2 and P_3 in a patient with P_2 prolapse. The figure 9C shows a 3 D transesophageal representation (surgical view) of a pseudo-cleft located between the P_3 and P_2 scallops (red arrow).

2.4.8 The pattern of 'floppy mitral valve'

Represents a redundant mitral valve, usually with both leaflet prolapse. It represents an excessive valve leaflet remodelling, with a 'finger like' transformation of the valve fabrics (Figure 10).

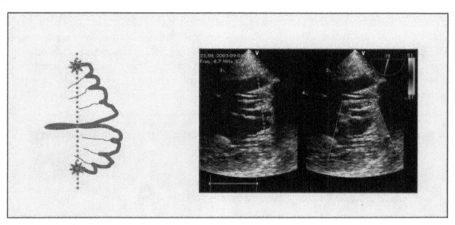

Fig. 10. Transgastric transesophageal intraoperative view of a 'floppy' mitral valve (zoom). Notice the extensive remodelling of the leaflet fabric.

2.4.9 The pattern of 'billowing mitral valve'

Is represented by the protrusion of the leaflet body into the left atrium cavity. As a rule, the coaptation point still remains into the left ventricular cavity (Figure 11). associated with mitral insufficiency, but it is important to indicate it to the surgical team.

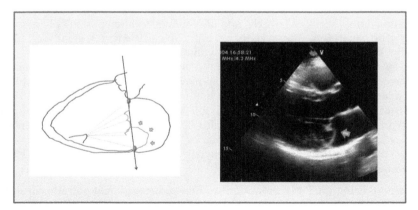

Fig. 11. Billowing mitral valve. PSLAx view of transthoracic exam showing the protrusion of the posterior leaflet (P_2 scallop) into the left atrial cavity. Often the mitral regurgitation may be absent or mild due to a pretty good coaptation, with the coaptation point still sited into the left ventricular cavity.

The final echo report contains coaptation height for each pair of scallops. The assessment of the triangle of coaptation, coaptation length and coaptation height. It represents an integrative scheme which is the synthesis of the various abnormalities found in different areas of the valve (Figure 1).

The mitral annular diameter must be assessed in parasternal long axis view. This measurement corresponds to the septo-marginal diameter of the valve, which is the most important diameter of mitral valve, because the mitral leaflets work in an anterior-posterior plane. The folding of the mitral leaflets depends on this diameter and not on the intercommissural diameter (Figure 12). Keep in mind that the TEE intraoperative measurement of the mitral annulus tends to underestimate it, due to intraoperative hypovolemic status and reduced overload.

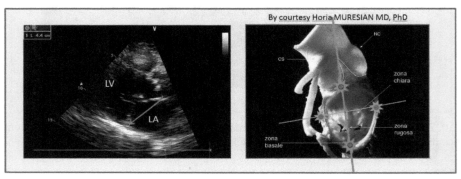

Fig. 12. Correct measurement of the mitral valve annulus in PSLAX view. This diameter corresponds to the septo-marginal diameter of the valve (red diameter on the anatomical photo). The intercommissural diameter (the green diameter in the photo) has to be avoided in the algorithm of decision for surgical planning.

The left ventricular dimensions (as EDØ and EDVolume) and function (LVEF) completes the diagnostic echo algorithm. The severity of mitral insufficiency is mainly quantitatively assessed by calculating the regurgitating volume using the PISA method (proximal isovelocity surface area) and vena contracta. Naturally, all other cardiac structures are carefully described, focusing on associated valvular lesions, mainly on the tricuspide valve. A special attention is paid to the left atrial volume, which may predict atrial fibrillation when measuring around 100ml as volume, or 50mm in diameter (parasternal long axis view). The preoperative assessment should also be focused to identify the patients at high risk to develop postoperative systolic anterior motion: hypertrophic interventricular septum, small left ventricular cavity, hyper dynamic left ventricle (see also 2.6.1 Prepump examination).

The final report, using the Prolapsing Score and the structured anatomical analysis focused on mitral geometry, allows the surgeon to be aware of the complexity of the lesions and to develop a tailored surgical strategy of repair. In general, the surgical strategy aims to correct mitral regurgitation with a single orifice (achieving a coaptation length of at least 6mm) and, whenever possible, to rebuild the triangle of coaptation by using the PTFE GoreTex chordae and annuloplasty.

The transthoracic echocardiography is almost always sufficient to select the patient candidate to mitral valve repair or replacement. The preoperative transesophageal exam serves to refine the diagnosis, mainly in terms of pseudo-commissures, commissural prolapse, ruptured chordae etc. It is mandatory and the only tool used to assess the outcome of surgery in postoperative period. The transesophageal three-dimensional echocardiography is the best tool in assessing the commissural lesions pre and postoperatively. Thus, the echocardiography is an essential tool in the assessment of mechanism of mitral regurgitation and in choosing the right timing and the proper planning for surgical repair. The surgical strategy is tailored by the prolapsing score and the structural echocardiographic algorithm. The successful repair of mitral valve requires a skilled team: an expert surgeon in valve repair and a dedicated echocardiographer.

2.5 Rebuilding the geometry of the mitral valve: Triangle of coaptation and coaptation length

Generally, the main target of the mitral valve repair is to achieve a minimum of 6mm of coaptation length. Initially, although not specified, this measure referred to the medial corresponding scallops A_2-P_2. As said before, the triangle of coaptation resembles an asymmetrical tent, meaning that the coaptation length varies among different regions of the valve. This fact was intuitive until recently, when studies were available in regard to the definition of the normal values of the coaptation for each valve region. Once three-dimensional echocardiography became available, this type of analysis was possible exclusively on an automatic base.

A recent study has defined the normal values of the coaptation length; these results indicated that the normal coaptation length in zone 1° (corresponding to the scallops A_1/P_1) is about 3.5mm; in zone 2° (scallops A_2/P_2) the coaptation length is round 6.2mm and finally in zone 3° (scallops A_3/P_3) the coaptation length seems to be slightly inferior to zone 1°, around 3.2mm. The authors also indicated that the contribution at coaptation of the anterior and posterior leaflets is not symmetrical. The anterior leaflet seems to have a major involvement compared to the posterior one in all the regions of the valve. This underlines the importance of the functional reserve of the anterior leaflet (Gogoladze, 2011).

Another recent study has proposed a new measure for the coaptation length, namely the coaptation length index, which represents the ratio between the coaptation length and the end-systolic annular septal-lateral diameter (Shudo, 2010). Lately, echocardiographic indexation of all measures (generally to the BSA), has gained much consideration. From this perspective, the new index looks promising but needs further investigation in order to establish its real practical value.

2.6 Evaluation of mitral regurgitation

Doppler echocardiography is the most common technique used for detection and evaluation of severity of valvular regurgitation. Several indexes have been used to assess the severity of regurgitation. The following paragraphs will make a brief description of the main indexes used in clinical practice, with their advantages and limitations. Surgery is addressed to patients with severe mitral degenerative regurgitation, and the quantification of the mitral insufficiency is a crucial point in the algorithm of decision. In the case of moderate mitral insufficiency, the surgery is considered only in patients with ischemic mitral regurgitation.

2.6.1 Proximal isovelocity surface area (PISA) or flow convergence

In most patients, PISA was the method of choice for the quantification of mitral regurgitation. As already extensively described, the PISA method is derived from the hydrodynamic principle stating that, as blood approaches a regurgitant orifice, its velocity increases, forming concentric roughly hemispheric shells of increasing velocity and decreasing surface area.

Colour flow mapping offers the ability to visualise one of these hemispheres that corresponds to the Nyquist limit of the instrument. If a Nyquist limit can be chosen at which the flow convergence becomes hemispheric in shape, the flow rate through the regurgitant orifice (ml/s) may be calculated as the product of the surface area of the hemisphere and the aliasing velocity. Assuming that the maximal PISA radius occurs at the time of peak regurgitant flow and peak regurgitant velocity, the maximal EROA is derived. The regurgitant volume can be estimated as EROA multiplied by the velocity time integral of the regurgitant jet. Since the PISA calculation provides an instantaneous peak flow rate, EROA by this approach is the maximal EROA and may be slightly larger than EROA calculated by other methods (Bargiggia, 1991).

As indicated by the guidelines of evaluation of valve regurgitation, the measurement of PISA by Colour Flow Mapping was done by adjustment of the aliasing velocity until a well-defined hemisphere was apparent. This was generally done by shifting the baseline towards the direction of flow, by lowering the Nyquist limit, or both. This has been shown to improve the reliability of the measurement (Zoghbi, 2003).

Despite the fact that it became the preferred method for evaluation of mitral regurgitation, the PISA method is far from being perfect. As with any other technique, limitations exist, e.g.: it is more accurate for central jets than for eccentric jets and for regurgitation with a circular orifice. If the image resolution allows a good visualisation of the flow convergence, and a Nyquist limit can be chosen in order to obtain a hemispheric shape of the convergence, it is easy to identify the aliasing line of the hemisphere. However, it can be difficult to judge the precise location of the orifice and the flow convergence shape. Any error introduced is then squared, which can markedly affect the resulting flow rate and EROA. Attention should be paid to remain as parallel as possible with the Doppler beam. In every day practice, the main error in grading the mitral insufficiency occurs with the eccentric jets. Fig 13 (A,B).

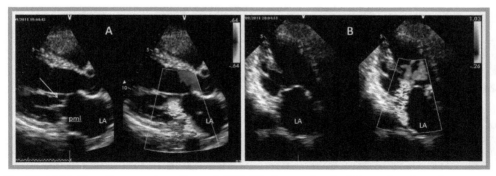

Fig. 13. (A,B). Simultaneous transthoracic PSLAX view and apical three chamber view showing an eccentric regurgitant jet in anterior mitral prolapse.

2.6.2 Color flow mapping

Mitral regurgitation has been most frequently evaluated through the Colour Doppler method. As all the guidelines use echocardiographic criteria to indicate surgery in valvular patients, the echocardiographer must be aware of the drawbacks of the echocardiographic criteria used to send the patients in the operating room.

For example, the maximal jet area correlates well with the semi quantitative angiographic grade of severity. However, only limited correlation is observed with quantitative measures of regurgitant volume and fraction. In addition, maximal jet area is not predictive of hemodynamic abnormalities, such as an elevated pulmonary capillary wedge pressure or reduced forward stroke volume. The regurgitant jet geometry, the physiologic variability, and the instrument settings are presumably some of the factors that may explain this reduced correlation with angiography.

Given the three-dimensional shape of the regurgitant flow, in all scanning sections, the regurgitant jet area will depend on the geometry and direction of the jet. Colour flow Doppler mapping of free regurgitant jets that are unbounded by surrounding structures may lead to overestimation of severity due to entrainment of adjacent fluid by the high-velocity jet. In contrast, the area of an eccentric jet is only 40% of the area of a free jet with the same regurgitant fraction. Eccentric jets are influenced by adjacent constraining surfaces, so that area measurements correlate poorly with regurgitant volume. It is also important to remember that the colour flow map of a regurgitant jet represents the spatial distribution of velocities and is not a direct measure of volume flow rate. Although colour Doppler jet area increases with regurgitant volume, this relationship is not linear because it is highly influenced by driving pressure, compliance of the receiving chamber, and the size and shape of the regurgitant orifice (Otto, 2002).

2.6.3 Vena contracta

It is one of the preferred echocardiographic indexes for its efficacy and its simplicity. The vena contracta is the narrowest portion of a jet that occurs at or just downstream from the orifice (Baumgartner, 1991). It is characterized by high velocity, laminar flow and is slightly smaller than the anatomic regurgitation orifice due to boundary effects.

The cross-sectional area of the vena contracta represents a measure of the effective regurgitant orifice area (EROA), which is the narrowest area of the actual flow. The size of the vena contracta is independent of the flow rate and driving pressure for a fixed orifice. However, if the regurgitant orifice is dynamic, the vena contracta may change with hemodynamics or during the cardiac cycle. Comprised of high velocities, the vena contracta is considerably less sensitive to technical factors such as PRF compared to the jet in the receiving chamber. To specifically image the vena contracta, it is often necessary to angulate the transducer out of the normal echocardiographic imaging planes, such that the area of proximal flow acceleration, the vena contracta, and the downstream expansion of the jet can be distinguished. It is preferable to use a zoom mode to optimize visualization of the vena contracta and facilitate its measurement. The Colour flow sector should also be as narrow as possible, with the minimal depth, so as to maximize lateral and temporal resolution.

Because of the small values of the width of the vena contracta (usually <1cm), small errors in its measurement may lead to a large percentage error and misclassification of the severity of regurgitation. Therefore, it is very important to acquire accurate primary data and measurement (Zoghbi, 2003).

The vena contracta method for assessing mitral regurgitation by colour Doppler echocardiography overestimates true mitral regurgitant orifice, it is markedly influenced by flow rate and the ultrasound system that is used. However, a diameter of a vena contracta over 8mm has a very good sensitivity and specificity for discriminating severe from non-severe mitral regurgitation (Zoghbi, 2003). The estimation of the diameter of the vena contracta is considered to have a good reproducibility of 10-15% (Margulescu, Brickner).

2.7 Intraoperative assessment of mitral regurgitation

The intraoperative echocardiography may be performed using the transesophageal or sometimes the epicardial method. In our practice we used almost exclusively the former. The epicardial approach may be used in paediatric cardiac surgery, when the adult TEE probe is too large and the paediatric TEE probe is not available.

2.7.1 Prepump examination

During the intraoperative transesophageal echocardiography, the evaluation of the severity of mitral regurgitation should be performed following the same steps and methodology as in all other echocardiographic examinations. It was observed that the degree of mitral regurgitation assessed by TEE in the operating theatre appears less severe in respect to the transthoracic exam. The team (anaesthesiologist, cardiologist and surgeon) has to be aware of the complexity of the changes induced by the general anaesthesia and the opening of the thorax and pericardial cavity. It also needs to be taken into account the loading condition of the heart, in term of the preload and afterload. Therefore, prepump TEE examination should not be used to assess the severity of the regurgitation, but mainly to assess its mechanism and the valve anatomy.

Important items on the preoperative echocardiographic check-list are the valve anatomy and the analysis of the coaptation: Does it exists? Is it absent or only reduced? In what valve sector is the coaptation missing or reduced? Why? Is there a prolapsed valve or flail? How much does each segment prolapse in regard to the mitral annular plane?

The answer to these final questions is essential for the surgeon who needs to perform a mitral valve repair. The correct evaluation of the entity of prolapse in tele-systole and in all segments may assist the surgeon in the decision of the length and position of the Gore-Tex neochordae they might need to use in order to correct the prolapse. In the operating theatre, the echocardiographer should measure the distance between the free border of the prolapsing scallop and the mitral annulus plane or the free border of the non-prolapsing scallop (Fig 14). This may be of great importance in measuring the length of the artificial chordae, but the experience of the surgeon remains the most important factor that will determine the final result.

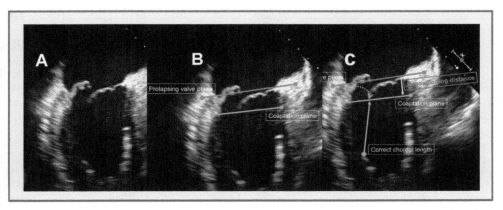

Fig. 14. (A,B,C). Intraoperative echocardiographic measurements showing prolapsed with flail of the posterior mitral leaflet (14A). The red line indicates the prolapsing plane; the green indicates the targeted coaptation plane (14B). Measuring the distance between the targeted position of the P2 scallop plane and the tip of the papillary muscle helps the surgeon decide the length of the neochordae (14C).

The preoperative echocardiographic examination must be performed under normal or near normal loading conditions. If hypovolemia were present, not only the severity of mitral regurgitation might be underestimated, as stated before, but also a false prolapse of various segments might erroneously be described. Often, a false prolapse may be encountered at the level of the anterior mitral leaflet (scallops A_2 and A_3) when, in fact, the lesion, usually flail, eversion or extreme prolapse, is typically located on the posterior leaflet. In order to avoid this risk, the echocardiographer should bear in mind the diagnosis of the preoperative transthoracic examination and carefully compare it to his own findings. One should not forget that most of the times the transesophageal examination confirms most of the elements from the transthoracic exam. By using the new harmonics echocardiographic machines, approximately 2/3 of the lesions found in transthoracic examination will be confirmed by TEE exam. The mitral annulus might also be underestimated when hypovolemia is present. This is the case in the operating room when the prepump exam is performed. In our experience the transthoracic measurement of the mitral annulus should always be taken into account when the surgical strategy is discussed with the surgeon.

It is important to remember that mitral regurgitation is dynamic and is affected by loading conditions. Reduction of afterload or intravascular volume at the time of the operation may reduce the true severity of the regurgitation. When mitral regurgitation is less significant than expected, the intravascular blood volume should be expanded and systemic vascular resistance should transiently be increased, by using repeated boluses of IV phenylephrine. The velocity of mitral regurgitation, and therefore display of its jet by Colour Doppler, depends on the pressure difference between the left atrium and left ventricle, which is higher in the presence of hypertension. The size of the jet in the left atrium is also very sensitive to changes in colour gain (directly proportional) and pulse repetition frequency (PRF) (inversely proportional). In any case, remember that the true assessment of the degree of mitral regurgitation is done by transthoracic exam.

The use of three-dimensional echocardiography for the evaluation of the mitral valve disease is rapidly evolving, especially in conjunction with the transesophageal echocardiography. One of the explanations of this extensive use is that the mitral valve rends itself to detailed 3D imaging from the left atrial perspective, as viewed by the surgeon (Shah & Raney, 2011). In our experience, three-dimensional echocardiography allows a reliable 'volumetric' evaluation with an excellent perspective on the whole mitral valve complex. Moreover, it permits an accurate (even more than the 2D echo) localisation of the various lesions. Still, the resolution and quality of the 3D images do not match those of the 2D echo.

2.7.2 Prepump examination: Risk of systolic anterior motion

Another important mission of the prepump examination is the identification of patients at risk for systolic anterior motion (SAM) of the anterior leaflet and subsequent functional mitral regurgitation. Fig 15 (A,B,C). The selection of patients at risk for SAM is already possible with the transthoracic approach. These patients usually have a small and /or hyper dynamic left ventricle, hypertrophy of the inter-ventricular septum, large posterior mitral leaflet, small mitral annulus and "narrow" LVOT (revealed by a reduced distance between the inter-ventricular septum and the coaptation line). One elegant study has indicated which could be the two echocardiographic indexes that may identify the patients at risk for SAM after surgery: the first is the ratio between the anterior and the posterior mitral leaflet (AL/PL) inferior to 1.3; the second is the distance from the coaptation line to the inter-ventricular septum (C-Sept) equal or inferior to 2.5cm. (Maslow, 1999).

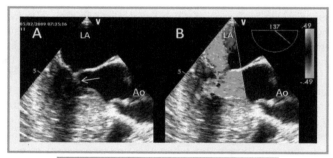

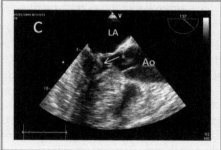

Fig. 15. (A,B,C). Postoperative transesophageal 2D exam showing the presence of SAM at the level of the anterior mitral leaflet (15 A, C, arrow) and the presence of severe mitral regurgitation (15 B).

For this category of patients, in order to avoid SAM, the surgeon must be informed and aware of each element stated above (e.g. hypertrophic septum associated or not with large posterior leaflet and / or small mitral annulus etc) and the surgical approach should be tailored accordingly. If SAM should appear, its management consists of volume expansion, withdrawal of positive inotropic agents and sometimes use of short acting betablockers like esmolol. However, there is one type of SAM which is irreversible, having a 'surgical mechanism': in case of large P_2 quadrangular resection without sliding plasty. This situation calls for a second run pump, to perform the sliding. This is particularly why the echocardiographer has to be aware of the surgical technique in the given case.

Left ventricular outflow tract obstruction caused by SAM has been described as a complication of mitral repair. It has generally been attributed to the implantation of an annuloplasty ring or to various surgical techniques that alter the normal systolic narrowing of the antero-posterior diameter of the mitral annulus, or due to the displacing the mitral coaptation level towards the interventricular septum. The period immediately after cardiopulmonary bypass is the most crucial time for the development of SAM. This is due to reduced peripheral vascular resistance associated with hypovolemia and hypotension, which have a particular impact when the left ventricular cavity is small. This adverse effect is determined by a hyper dynamic state (increased kinetic energy of blood flow induced by catecholamines), associated with left ventricular hypovolemia.

Mild degrees of LVOT dynamic obstruction after mitral valve repair often respond favourably to conservative treatment, as stated before: discontinuing inotropic agents in order to decrease contractility and heart rate, volume loading to increase preload, and augmenting afterload with pure α-agonists (such as phenylephrine) (Benea, 2005). If these measures prove inadequate, reoperation upon the mitral valve — including the performance of a sliding plasty or folding reconstruction that reduces the antero-posterior height of the posterior leaflet, the implantation of an annuloplasty ring of a larger size or the removal of the annuloplasty ring — may prove necessary. In refractory cases, even prosthetic mitral valve replacement has been reported.

2.7.3 Tailored surgical strategy

Based on the Prolapsed Score and on the structured echocardiographic analyses of the mitral valve, the surgical strategy has to be personalised. In order to choose the right surgical approach and to be able to interact with the surgeon, the echocardiographer needs to know the surgical techniques suitable for the given case. Building a trust-based relationship between the surgeon and the echocardiographer is crucial for the surgical result. Each case has to be discussed by the surgical team prior to the operation.

This approach allows the surgeon to make two types of surgical planning, both necessary: one is the planning with 'the closed atrium', meaning the mental planning based on the echocardiographic findings. The other one is performed after the left atrium was opened and the valve is directly inspected. In our experience the two coincide in most of the cases, due to standardization of the echo exam, to the presence of the echocardiographer in the operating room and due to the dialogue with the surgical team.

Recently, the importance of performing the mitral valve repair using the most 'physiological' approach has become crucial. Single valve orifice but also posterior mitral leaflet mobility became cornerstone principles that guide the mitral repair in our centre. The classical techniques of repair included the quadrangular resection of the posterior mitral leaflet and ring annuloplasty, which inevitably led to a rigid posterior leaflet (Verma, NYJM 2009). Lately, many surgeons have chosen to perform the triangular resection (instead of quadrangular) in order to guarantee a higher mobility of the posterior leaflet and thus an increased anatomical and functional leaflet reserve, convinced that this will subsequently achieve a better and longer lasting coaptation.

In conclusion, we may assume that the importance of the preoperative transesophageal examination is given by the accuracy in identifying the mechanism of mitral regurgitation and valve anatomy (flail, prolapse, loss of coaptation, perforation and so on), and by describing the geometry of the mitral apparatus. There is a close correlation between valve geometry and function. The Colour Doppler mapping might underestimate the entity of the regurgitant flow; thus, the prepump echocardiographic evaluation needs to rely more on valve geometry and regurgitant mechanism, and less on the Colour flow Doppler.

2.7.4 Postpump examination

In most cases, with an experienced surgeon, mitral valve repair leads to a competent mitral valve with mild or no residual mitral regurgitation. However, there are potential complications of mitral valve repair that are readily recognized by postpump intraoperative echocardiography. Many of these complications may not be apparent clinically or may take longer to accurately diagnose without echocardiography. If left untreated, these complications may interfere with the long-term success of the procedure and require early re-operation (Otto, 2003). In fact, the trust-based relationship between the echocardiographer and the surgeon is tested when a second run pump is needed. In case of debatable "moderate" mitral regurgitation, the team has to focus on the mitral coaptation (and geometry) rather than on the Colour Doppler analyses. Remember to avoid the hypovolemic status.

Transesophageal echocardiography is practically the only method used immediately after weaning from the cardiopulmonary bypass in order to assess the result of the mitral repair. It must rapidly answer some essential questions about the repaired valve. The most important task of the transesophageal echocardiography is to analyze the postoperative mitral valve geometry and function, focusing on leaflet coaptation.

 It may occur that immediately after weaning the patient off the cardiopulmonary by-pass, the echocardiographer declares the success of the repair after analyzing only some of the available views, usually the mid-esophageal 0° or distal-esophageal 135°, where only scallops A_2 and P_2 are evaluated. The postoperative transesophageal examination has to be performed using the same algorithm that was used during the preoperative evaluation. One has to bear in mind that the triangle of coaptation remains the goal of a typically functioning reconstructed valve. It should be taken into consideration that the reconstruction of the coaptation triangle is not always possible. When present, the echocardiographer has to search for it in all the segments of the valve: from the anterior commissure and corresponding scallops A_1/P_1, P_2/A_2 and of course the medial scallops A_3/P_3 and the posterior commissure.

After surgical repair, the essential issue is that the coaptation point must be dragged within the left ventricle, underneath the mitral annular plane (Figure 15). In the normal mitral valve, this type of coaptation expresses the physiological equilibrium between the collagen and elastic fibres, which confers the right balance between the elasticity and resistance of the valve. Same should be true about the repaired mitral valves, which will most probably remain elastic and long-lasting when their geometry satisfies the mentioned criteria.

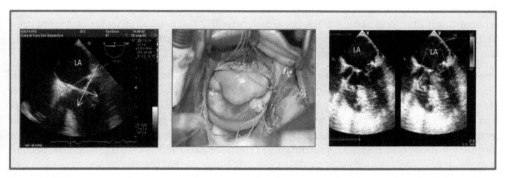

Fig. 16. TEE postoperative aspect of complex mitral valve repair. Notice the rebuilding of the triangle of coaptation (arrows) and the classical 'smile' aspect of the mitral valve on the intraoperative photo (middle). LA = left atrium.

Even if already stated, it should be underlined that the triangle of coaptation and the coaptation length need to be carefully assessed in all the regions of the mitral valve before expressing the final judgement on the real immediate outcome of the repair. Keep in mind possible traps. The surgeon's "hurry" to know the results of repair; do not express any conclusions before appropriate ventricular loading conditions are achieved. Do not start the post-operative assessment by Colour Doppler. The most important thing is to assess the length of coaptation and valve geometry.

In order to correctly assess the valve geometry, the loading conditions should be optimal: hypovolemia should be avoided as it may underestimate a potential residual mitral regurgitation or label as 'prolapsing' an otherwise normal valve leaflet. We have stated about the prepump exam that the importance of the Doppler techniques for the evaluation of the severity of the mitral regurgitation was lower than the importance of the geometrical analysis. This does not mean that Color Doppler mapping shouldn't be performed but it should integrate the geometrical analysis and not replace it. These details are essential to the surgeon. The outcome depends on that. This statement is also true about the post-pump examination. Geometry is more important than colour (meaning Colour Doppler mapping).

Whenever the result of the repair is suboptimal and there is residual mitral regurgitation, the echocardiographer must be able to rapidly identify the true mechanism of mitral regurgitation. The problem may vary from residual prolapse or restriction of one or more valve sectors - presumably due to incorrect neo-cordal length, residual marginal prolapse if left untreated, oversized annuloplasty ring, persistence of pseudo-commissures, etc. In these cases further surgery with a second run pump might be needed. Rarely, the mitral valve problem may be a consequence of a ventricular dysfunction when a post-pump contractility issue may appear. This should also be clearly pointed out by the post-pump echocardiographic examination. In this case, further surgery for the mitral valve might not be needed, but only ventricular assistance.

The main problem with residual mitral regurgitation arises in patients with moderate insufficiency. In loose teams, the surgeon tends to underestimates the importance of the mitral regurgitation. Because the echocardiography is a semi quantitative method, in every day practice the surgeon will go easier to the second run pump only if the echocardiographer was able to 100% accurately identify the preoperative lesions, compared to the intraoperative findings. Therefore, an excellent preoperative assessment will bond the team, creating a trustful relationship between the surgeon and the echocardiographer.

The evaluation of the outcome after mitral repair has been done mainly using the Colour Doppler mapping. When the residual regurgitation is absent or of mild degree, the result is judged as adequate. Generally, superior degrees of residual regurgitation, naturally correlated with the coaptation and geometrical analysis, indicate the need for a second pump run. In selected cases (e.g. old patients or significant comorbidities), moderate or more than moderate residual regurgitation might be accepted when the risk of a second pump run to correct the valvular problem exceeds the potential benefit for the patient.

The annuloplasty ring is used in almost all operated patients. From an echocardiographic technical perspective this might determine difficulties in the postoperative evaluation of the repaired mitral valve when performing the distal esophageal long axis views. Usually, the presence of the annuloplasty ring might 'hide' the mitral valve leaflets by posterior shadowing immediately after surgery. To overcome this problem a valid solution could be the evaluation from the deep transgastric short-axis and long axis views.

3. Conclusion

The standardization of the preoperative, intraoperative and postoperative echocardiographic examination is crucial for the skilled dialogue with the surgical team and for the results. As the surgery of degenerative mitral insufficiency is somehow standardised, echocardiography should also be as standardised as possible. The use of a specific pattern of lesion confers better and tailored surgical planning, adapted to each given case. Use of different types of patterns such as mitral valve flail, undulating valve or marginal prolapse facilitates the dialog with the surgeon.

Alongside specific patterns of lesions, a crucial point in surgical repair is the evaluation of the mitral geometry. Apart from the three dimensional echo, the main tool in assessing the mitral valve geometry by 2 D echocardiography, is the coaptation triangle.

The echocardiographer must consider the mitral valve as an eight-element anatomical structure, and separately assess each segment. The preoperative exam has to be done based on a structural echocardiographic algorithm and finally expressed as a prolapsing score.

By using this strategy, the mitral valve repair is feasible, with excellent results.

In dedicated centres, the mitral valve repair for degenerative disease is possible with more than 95% rate of success. The use of the triangle of coaptation, coaptation length and coaptation height as geometric echocardiographic concepts aiming to restore the mitral valve shape and coaptation, is a crucial point to improve the surgical planning and results.

4. Acknowledgements

We acknowledge BENEA Diana MD and IONESCU Georgiana MD, for helpful contribution to the manuscript.

5. References

Bargiggia, GS.; Tronconi, L.; Sahn, DJ.; Recusani, F.; Raisaro, A. & De Servi, S. A new method for quantitation of mitral regurgitation based on color flow Doppler imaging of flow convergence proximal to regurgitant orifice. *Circulation.* Vol 84. No 4 (October 1991); pp. 1481-9, ISSN 1524-4539.

Baumgartner, H.; Schima, H. & Kuhn, P.; Value and limitations of proximal jet dimensions for the quantitation of valvular regurgitation: an in vitro study using Doppler flow imaging. *Journal of the American Society of Echocardiography*, Vol 4, (Jan-Feb 1991), pp. 57-66

Benea, D.; Cerin, G.; Diena, M. & Tesler, UF. Pharmacologic Resolution of Functional Out flow Tract Obstruction after Mitral Valve Repair. *Texas Heart Institute Journal*, Vol 32, No 4. (October 2005), pp. 563–566, ISSN 0730-2347

Bonow, R. (2011). Valvular heart disease: Patient needs and practice guidelines. *Aswan Heart Center Science & Practice Series*, Vol 1 (April 2011), pp. 20-29, ISSN 2220-2730

Brickner ME, Willet DL, Irani WN-Assesement of Mitral RegurgitationSeverity by Doppler Color Flow Mapping of the Vena Contracta. Circulation 1997;95:636-642

G Cerin, M Diena, G Lanzillo, S Casalino, A Zito, D Benea, U Filippo Tesler. Degenerative mitral regurgitation - surgical and echocardiographic consideration for repair. Romanian Journal of Cardiovascular Surgery, 5 (3), pp. 131-39, 2006.

Cerin, G.; Popa, BA.; Benea, D.; Lanzillo, G.; Karazanishvili, L.; Casati, V.; Popa, A.; Novelli, E.; Renzi, L. & Diena, M. The triangle of coaptation: a new concept to enhance mitral valve repair through reshaping the native geometry. *World Congress of Cardiology Scientific Sessions*, Beijing, China (June 2010)

Gogoladze, G.; Dellis, SL.; Donnino, R.; Ribakove, G.; Greenhouse, DG.; Galloway, A. & Grossi E. (April 2011). Analysis of the mitral coaptation zone in normal and functional regurgitant valves. *The Annals of Thoracic Surgery*, Vol 89, Issue 4, pp. 1158-1161

Hall SA, Brickner ME, Willett DL, Irani WN, Afridi I, Grayburn PA – Assessment of Mitral Regurgitation Severity by Doppler Color Flow Mapping of the Vena Contracta. Circulation. 1997; 95:636-642).

Maslow, DA.; Regan, MM.; Haering, MJ.; Johnson, RG. & Levine RA(1999). Echocardiographic predictors of left ventricular outflow tract obstruction and systolic anterior motion of the mitral valve after mitral valve reconstruction for myxomatous valve disease. *Journal of the American College of Cardiology*, Vol 37, No 7, (December 1999), pp. 2096-2104, ISSN 0735-1097

Mirabel, M; Iung,B, Baron, G; Messika-Zeitoun, D & Détaint, D. Surgical referral in symptomatic mitral regurgitation: greater compliance with guidelines is needed *European Heart Journal* 2007, 28, 1358-1365

Jean-Louis Vanoverschelde, Eric G. Butchart, Philippe Ravaud and Alec Vahanian. What are the characteristics of patients with severe, symptomatic, mitral regurgitation who are denied surgery? Euro Heart J 2007, 28, 1358-1365

Margulescu, AD; Cinteza, M & Vinereanu, D (2006). Reproducibility in echocardiography: clinical significance, assessment, and comparison with other imaging methods. *Mædica A Journal of Clinical Medicine*, Vol 1, No 7, (2006), ISSN1841-9038

Otto, C. (2002) *The Practice of Clinical Echocardiography, 2nd Edition*, W. B. Saunders Company, ISBN 0-7216-9204-4, Philadelphia, USA

Shah, PM. & Raney, AA. Impact of 3D echocardiography on mitral valve surgery. *Aswan Heart Center Science & Practice Series*, Vol 1 (April 2011), pp. 36-44, ISSN 2220-2730

Shudo, Y.; Matsue, H.; Toda, K.; Hata, H.; Fujita, S.; Taniguchi, K. & Sawa, Y. A simplified echocardiographic measurements of direct effects of restrictive annuloplasty on mitral valve geometry. *Echocardiography*, Vol 27, No 8, (September 2010), pp. 931-936, ISSN 0742-2822

Tesler, UF.; Cerin, G.; Novelli, E.; Popa, A. & Diena, M. Evolution of surgical techniques for mitral valve repair. *Texas Heart Institute Journal*, Vol 36, No 5. (November 2009), pp. 438-4, ISSN 0730-2347

Subodh Verma, and Thierry G. Mesana, Mitral-Valve Repair for Mitral-Valve Prolapse. N Engl J Med 2009; 361:2261-9.

Zoghbi, A. et al (2003). Recommendations for evaluation of the severity of native valvular regurgitation with two-dimensional and Doppler echocardiography. *Journal of the American Society of Echocardiography*. Vol. 16, No 7, (July 2003), pp. 777-802, ISSN 0894-7317

3

Epiaortic Ultrasound Assessment of the Thoracic Aorta in Cardiac Surgery

Alistair Royse[1] and Colin Royse[2]
[1]Department of Surgery, and
[2]Pharmacology, The University of Melbourne,
The Royal Melbourne Hospital
Australia

1. Introduction

A considerable burden of cerebral embolism in association with cardiac surgery reflects dislodgement of aortic atheroma caused by manipulating the aorta during a surgical procedure (Barbut and Gold 1996; Van Zaane, Zuithoff et al. 2008; Whitley and Glas 2008; Yamaguchi, Adachi et al. 2009). It clearly makes logical sense to identify and attempt to avoid dislodgement of aortic atheroma. This strategy depends on two key elements; the accurate detection of atheroma in the aorta, and the surgeons ability to avoid or otherwise minimise manipulation of atheromatous disease.

In this chapter we will describe how epiaortic echocardiography is essential to the complete examination of the ascending aorta and aortic arch for the detection of atheroma, and what surgical options may be available for the avoidance or minimisation of aortic atheroma manipulation.

2. Background summary of the literature

2.1 Intraoperative cerebral embolism and brain dysfunction

Whilst clinical stroke is relatively infrequent in cardiac surgery (1-3%) (Calafiore, Di Mauro et al. 2002; Douglas and Spaniol 2009; Rosenberger, Shernan et al. 2008; Shroyer, Coombs et al. 2003), such events can be properly viewed as major cerebral injury. Subclinical brain injury on the other hand is not often clinically apparent but may be detected by subtle neurocognitive testing and this is frequently present (20-60%) (Hammon, Stump et al. 1997; Mahanna, Blumenthal et al. 1996; Zamvar, Williams et al. 2002). MRI studies post cardiac surgery similarly highlight a far higher frequency of cerebral embolic events then the clinical assessment of neurological status would suggest (Deslauriers, Saunders et al. 1996; Djaiani, Fedorko et al. 2004; Vanninen, Aikia et al. 1998). Brain injury may be caused by other factors related to cardiopulmonary bypass, systemic inflammatory response syndrome, tissue oedema, air embolism, post-operative hypotension, anaesthetic agents used, ischaemia and reperfusion injury, or alternative causes of embolism. Nevertheless, the *predominant cause* of embolic brain injury reflects surgical manipulation of the atheromatous aorta and thus offers the greatest prospect for changing outcome.

2.2 Assessment of the aorta

Surgeons traditionally assess the aorta by manual palpation prior to the placement of the cannula and clamp. This is problematic because it relies on the detection of calcified plaques in the wall of the aorta that are accessible to the finger; which predominantly reflects the anterior and right sides of the ascending aorta, and anterior aspect of the aortic arch. Other areas of the aorta are really not accessible or not easily accessible to manual palpation. The detection of calcified plaques infers resistance being offered to the surgeon's finger, and our previous data found that detection of such plaques was relatively accurate under these circumstances. What are not accurately detected are soft (not calcified) plaques, which do not offer counter resistance to the examining finger. However the propensity of these to disrupt and embolise the contents or components is potentially greater than for calcified plaques. Thus the manual examination of the ascending aorta by the surgeon should be considered as frequently inaccurate (Royse, Royse et al. 2000; Royse, Royse et al. 1998; Suvarna, Smith et al. 2007; Sylivris, Calafiore et al. 1997; Whitley and Glas 2008).

Transoesophageal echocardiography is not able to visualise the distal ascending aorta or the proximal aortic arch. This is because the distal trachea and right main bronchus lie between oesophagus and these structures, and so the ultrasound signal is not transmitted leading to poor or absent imaging. Furthermore, the anterior aortic wall is further than near structures in relation to the probe, further diminishing resolution. Yet the most frequent locality for placement of the aortic cannula for cardiopulmonary bypass is in the distal ascending aorta proximal or aortic arch. Equally, the aortic clamp is placed immediately proximal to the aortic cannula whereby there is substantial aortic manipulation. Thus, the key areas of aortic manipulation related to the use of cardiopulmonary bypass occur in the "blind spot" of transoesophageal echocardiography.

This point was reinforced by a meta-anaylsis performed by van Zaane comparing transoesophageal vs. epiaortic echocardiography (Van Zaane, Zuithoff et al. 2008). Transoeosphageal had a sensitivity of only 21% (95% confidence interval (CI) 12-32%); but a specificity of 99% (95% CI 96-99%). Simply TOE is accurate at assessing the aorta that can be visualised, but not all of the aorta can be imaged. Therefore, the accurate assessment of all parts of the thoracic aorta require a combination of transoesophageal and epiaortic (epivascular) surface ultrasound.

2.3 The precise anatomical location of aortic atheroma

Of critical importance to the use of epiaortic ultrasound, is the ability to precisely locate atheroma in relation to anatomical landmarks. The use of TOE provides for relative anatomical locality by finding lesions relative to the locality of other landmarks seen, such as the aortic valve. TOE alone will therefore lead to imperfect localisation of the aortic atheroma; whereas use of a handheld probe provides definitive locality of aortic atheroma (since the lesion is present immediately beneath the probe). This is crucial when precise locality on cannulation or clamping is required in order to avoid atheroma.

2.4 Prevalence of thoracic aortic atheroma

Surprisingly, coronary bypass patients do not uniformly have aortic atheroma, even in the presence of extensive small vessel arterial disease. But the danger for surgeons (and patients) is assuming that the presence of important aortic atheroma is predictable. Indeed the unpredictability of the presence, location and severity of aortic atheroma is the most powerful argument in favor of routine comprehensive ultrasound examination of the entire thoracic aorta being performed. Specifically, the absence of atheroma seen in the descending aorta or proximal aorta by TOE does *not always predict* the absence of clinically important atheroma in the distal ascending aorta or proximal arch (the TOE "blind spot") (Royse, Royse et al. 1998).

We described six zones for the thoracic aorta; three in the ascending aorta, two in the aortic arch and the descending aorta. TOE typically images zones 1-2 and 5-6 well; and epiaortic echocardiography images zones 1-4 well. For reference, most aortic cannulations and clamping occurs in zones 3-4; proximal aortic graft anastomoses in zone 2 and aortic incision for valve replacements in zone 1. An intra-aortic balloon pump will be deployed in zone 6. Within these zones, the site of the atheroma is further subcategorised into cross sectional quadrants of the aorta - anterior, posterior, left or right lateral.

We found that the prevalence of atheroma increased with distance from the aortic root. There was a marked increase in frequency and severity distal to the aortic arch. Increasing age resulted in greater prevalence. Considering moderate or severe atheroma in zones 1-4, the prevalence was 29% in patients aged 70-79, and 34% in those aged more than 80 years (Royse and Royse 2006).

2.5 Assessment of aortic atheroma severity

A variety of definitions have been published, but most commonly this simple classification is used, Table 1 (Royse, Royse et al. 1998). The greater the severity of atheroma, the greater the likelihood that manipulation will result in embolism; excepting that most believe embolism is unlikely to arise from "mild" atheroma. In clinical practice the term "clinically important atheroma" generally refers to moderate or severe atheroma.

Grade	Criteria
Nil	Intimal thickening < 2 mm
Mild	Intimal thickening 2 – 4 mm
Moderate	Flat intimal thickening > 4 mm
Severe	Complex intimal thickening > 4 mm or any mobile atheroma

Table 1. Classification of atheroma grade

The morphology of the atheromatous plaque may further predict the likelihood of embolism. Without good data, it would seem intuitive that a soft friable, frond-like atheromatous plaque is more likely to break free and embolise, than a flat, fibrous plaque.

3. Strategies to avoid aortic atheroma dislogement

The detection of aortic atheroma does not directly lead to the avoidance of atheroma dislodgement and embolism. The actual avoidance of dislodgement requires a change to the surgical strategy. Thus the detection of atheroma is the important first step, and allows a decision to be made that then subsequently leads to the avoidance of embolism. This highlights one of the key difficulties for surgeons. It may be that a surgical alternative is not possible for the patient; or the skill, capability or surgical repertoire of the surgeon themselves limits potential alternative strategies being employed. This may vary with training, experience and technical capability as well as patient factors such as absence of suitable conduits and so forth. Thus there is no commonly applied solution available.

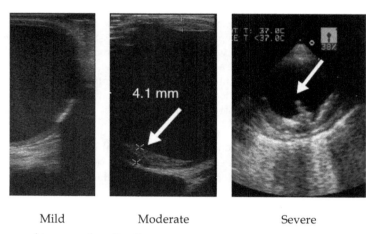

| Mild | Moderate | Severe |

Fig. 1. Ultrasound images of aortic atheroma.

In principle however, there are few significant options available for surgical alteration. In the case of the use of cardiopulmonary bypass, aortic calculation and clamping sites may be altered so as to manipulate the aorta near to but not involving the atheroma. Certain operations preclude alteration of manipulation position, and so alternative sites for aortic cannulation or alternatives for aortic clamping need to be considered. In practice, often the surgeon simply accepts the need to manipulate atheromatous segments of the aorta and proceeds anyway. An example may be the performance of an aortic valve replacement; whereby there is very limited scope for alteration of the aortic incision, and it may not be possible to entirely avoid atheroma in this locality.

Coronary artery bypass surgery provides more opportunity to alter the surgical operation so as to avoid atheroma. The construction of proximal aortic anastomoses is predominantly situated in the mid ascending aorta; the proximal aorta is rarely used as this will kink the grafts and the distal ascending aorta is occupied by the aortic clamp and antegrade cannula. So unless the grafting strategy is altered, the detection of aortic atheroma and the need to move the site of cannulation and clamping is impeded by the inability to move the proximal aortic anastomoses. By performing a composite graft (Y-graft), the aortic anastomoses can be eliminated, thereby allowing the freedom to move sites of aortic manipulation (Royse, Royse et al. 2000; Royse, Royse et al. 1999), see Fig. 2. Should there be extensive aortic atheroma, consideration of "off pump" coronary revascularisation would allow the complete avoidance of any aortic manipulation - the ideal solution from this perspective. Many surgeons however, are not comfortable or skilled in these techniques, thereby limiting their use.

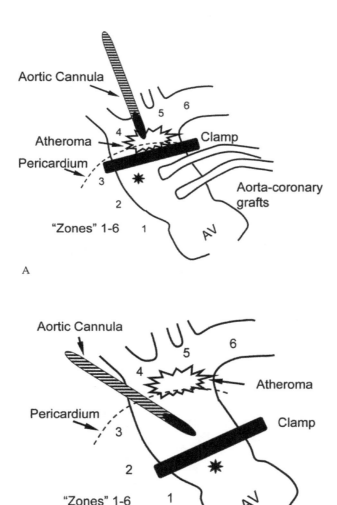

Fig. 2. Freedom to move sites of aortic manipulation. The sites of aortic manipulation are shown for (A) aorta-coronary and (B) Y graft techniques. Construction of aortic anastomosis limits movement of aortic cannulation and clamp sites away from detected atheroma illustrated in the distal ascending and proximal aortic arch. The atheroma is easily avoided by using the exclusive Y graft technique by moving the sites of cannulation and clamping away from the atheroma. (Small star (*) is antegrade cardioplegia cannulation site; AV is aortic valve.)

The technique of aortic clamping itself varies, with the repeated application of the aortic clamp rather than the "single clamp" technique; and use of the partial occlusion clamp for the construction of proximal aortic coronary anastomoses, further manipulates the aorta and will lead to greater propensity for dislodgement of any existing aortic atheroma. In particular, the typical Kaye-Lambert partial occlusion ("side biting") clamp will usually occupy the majority of the ascending aorta in a vertical plane and about half of the cross sectional diameter of the aorta in the horizontal plane, see Fig. 3. This clamp will therefore manipulate a considerable part of the ascending aorta even with only one application; and repeated applications would be common.

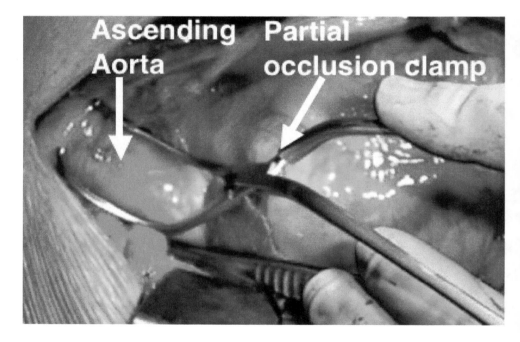

Fig. 3. Partial occlusion clamp manipulates most of the ascending aorta

4. Technique of epiaortic (epivascular) ultrasound examination

The sequence and technique have been previously published (Royse and Royse 2006) Fig. 4 or with Guidelines (Glas, Swaminathan et al. 2008). One important point to appreciate is that the orientation of the aorta to orthogonal planes is highly variable. For accurate cross-sectional dimensions, the ultrasound probe needs to be oriented at 90 degrees to the aorta irrespective of the relationship to the orthogonal plane, Fig. 5. This is not difficult to achieve, and it is obvious as you simply rotate the probe to produce a circle on the screen; yet it is a common failing in the early learning experience.

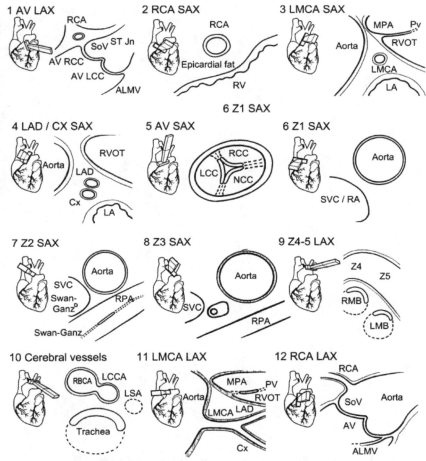

Fig. 4. Standardised epiaortic echocardiography examination. (Royse and Royse 2006)
Intraoperative ultrasound examination of the aorta and proximal coronary arteries 10 standard
views, 2 supplementary views. LAX, longitudinal axis, SAX, short axis, RCA, right coronary
artery, SoV, Sinus of Valsalva, AV, aortic valve, RCC, right coronary cusp of aortic valve, LCC,
left coronary cusp, NCC, non coronary cusp, ST Jn, sinotubular junction of aorta, ALMV,
anterior leaflet of mitral valve, RV, right ventricle, RVOT, right ventricular outflow tract, MPA,
main pulmonary artery, PV, pulmonary valve, LA, left atrium, LAD, left anterior descending
artery, Cx, circumflex coronary artery, SVC, superior vena cava, RA, right atrium, RPA, right
pulmonary artery, Z1, zone 1 or proximal ascending aorta, Z2, zone 2 or mid ascending, Z3,
zone 3 or distal ascending, Z4, zone 4 or proximal aortic arch, Z5, zone 5 or distal aortic arch,
RMB, right main bronchus, LMB, left main bronchus, RBCA, right brachiocephalic artery,
LCC, left common carotid artery, LSA, left subclavian artery. Reproduced from Royse A and
Royse C. A standardised intraoperative ultrasound examination of the aorta and proximal
coronary arteries. Interact CardioVasc Thorac Surg 2006;5:701-704. © 2006 European
Association of Cardio-Thoracic Surgery with permission from the European Association of
Cardio-Thoracic Surgery.

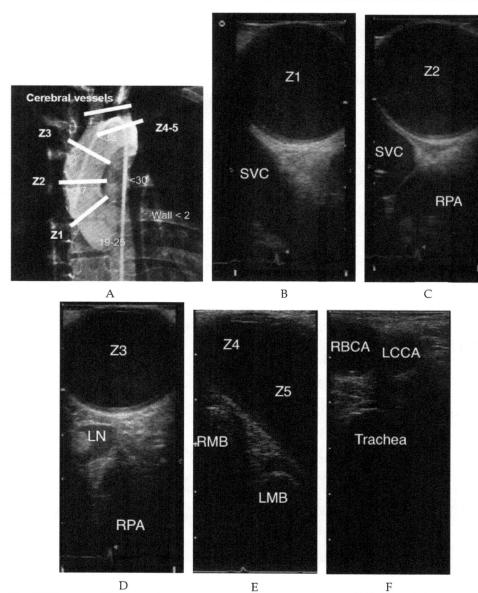

Fig. 5. Ultrasound images of aorta. A angles ot ultrasound probe. B Zone 1, C Zone 2, D Zone 3, E Aortic arch, F Cerebral vessels. Other abbreviations as for Fig. 4.Ultrasound probe selection is important. A phased, linear array probe with a frequency in the rage 8-12 Mhz is preferred. Some attention to the physical size is also important as a large probe may not easily fit in the sternotomy wound, and a round probe is difficult to hold or to maintain orientation. If the frequency is too high, then the depth of penetration may be sufficiently limited so as to preclude adequate imaging of the posterior aortic wall.

A variety of ways exist to allow a sterile acoustic interface for the probe. The simplest is to partially fill a sterile plastic cover with saline - either a custom made bag or a bag adapted from another use such as an endoscopic camera cover. Alternatively, sterile gel may be placed within the bag as the internal acoustic couple. Some fill the pericardium with warm saline to enhance the external acoustic couple; most do not. One important point that is often overlooked is the issue of "near field crowding". What this refers to is the need to maintain some distance between the ultrasound probe and the structure being imaged in order for the ultrasound to travel some distance, and then be reflected from the structure back to the probe. This is important for visualising the superficial (anterior) aortic wall. This wall cannot be adequately imaged when the probe is resting directly on the surface; and in order to adequately image this part of the aorta, the probe needs to be moved away from the aorta by 0.5-1.0 cm. Of course the acoustic coupling between the probe and the structure in question needs to be maintained, but generally this is not a problem when saline has been used within the plastic bag in which the probe is suspended.

There is no rationale or valid reason for any particular order or protocol to be followed whilst performing a study. However, it makes logical sense to follow a routine in order to efficiently complete a comprehensive study. See Fig. 4 for a proposed sequence. Special-purpose ultrasound examinations may be performed without the need for a comprehensive examination. One example may be to interrogate flow in the right coronary artery following an aortic valve replacement where there is some doubt as to whether the prosthesis was obstructing the flow to this coronary artery.

The operator performing the ultrasound examination is (or should be) the surgeon. The anaesthetist should be recording sample images or video loops as the examination is being performed so that appropriate archiving of the findings occurs. The fascinating thing about the subject of atheroma detection and this ultrasound examination is that very little new knowledge or new techniques have occurred in the past 10-15 years. The evidence is very strong that the performance of this study accurately establishes the presence and location of aortic atheroma and provides the surgeon with a greater range treatment options. Remarkably, this is not a routine part of every cardiac surgical procedure! Indeed only the minority of surgeons actually perform epiaortic ultrasound examinations and even fewer still, perform this on a routine basis.

5. Training

This ultrasound examination pertains almost exclusively to cardiac surgery. It could quite easily be applied to any other forms of surgery involving examination of large arteries or veins. At the current time intraoperative transoesophageal echocardiography is routine in many parts of the Western world, and becoming more common in the developing world. Therefore generally there is a good level of basic ultrasound experience and knowledge amongst surgical staff from the general observation of ultrasound being performed. However, at present few will be actively performing ultrasound examinations such as transthoracic echocardiography, ultrasound guided procedures or venous duplex studies all of which are becoming standard practice in advanced cardiac surgical centres. With this familiarity, the performance of epiaortic ultrasound examination is extremely simple to implement and to teach since there is significant underlying theoretical and practical experience. For those who have not performed ultrasound examinations before themselves;

or have quite limited theoretical knowledge of ultrasound technologies, learning this examination is a little more difficult. The emphasis here is on the word "little", highlighting that this examination is quite straightforward and simple to perform and therefore to learn. Also, interpreting the images is equally very simple since it is obvious from first principles without any formal training, and the precise locality of atheroma is similarly very easy to appreciate since it is always directly beneath the ultrasound probe at the time. Surgeons do not require additional anatomy training; indeed the level of anatomy knowledge is the greatest of all specialties and even trainees have an extremely good understanding of anatomy. It would be expected that an advanced surgical trainee should be able to competently and confidently perform and epiaortic ultrasound examination after about 10-20 supervised cases. With previous practical and theoretical experience in ultrasound or echocardiography, it may only be 5-10 cases.

Learning epiaortic ultrasound examination may be a sufficient enough stimulus to engage in a wider use of ultrasound technologies. In the current advanced cardiac surgical management, the use of ultrasound by cardiac surgeons should become a matter of routine daily practice. Performing transthoracic echocardiography in the pre-and post-operative settings, ultrasound guided procedures including pleural drainage and ultrasound lung examinations are quite straightforward and simple to learn. However, specific postgraduate training in addition to advanced surgical training should be undertaken; specifically it is not yet integrated as part of an advanced training program. A variety of postgraduate courses are available including university-based courses. These may cater for general (non-cardiac) clinical practice, or for an advanced diagnostic (cardiac) practice. Our program may be reviewed at www.heartweb.com

6. Summary and recommendations

The predominant cause for cerebral atheroma embolism in cardiac surgery using cardiopulmonary bypass relates to dislodgement of aortic atheroma with embolism caused by manipulation of the aorta. Transoesophageal echocardiography is not able to visualise the distal ascending aorta and proximal aortic arch due to the presence of air in the bronchi crossing between aorta and oesophagus. Epiaortic ultrasound is able to assess this portion of the aorta; and in addition is far more accurate than manual assessment by the surgeon's finger. Avoiding the atheroma however, requires a change to the surgical strategy.

A standardised comprehensive echocardiography protocol is proposed. The performance of this ultrasound examination is relatively straightforward and is fairly easily taught. It is recommended that it be before routinely.

7. References

Barbut, D.&J. P. Gold (1996). Aortic atheromatosis and risks of cerebral embolization. *J Cardiothorac Vasc Anesth* 10(1): 24-29.

Calafiore, A. M., M. Di Mauro, et al. (2002). Impact of aortic manipulation on incidence of cerebrovascular accidents after surgical myocardial revascularization. *Ann Thorac Surg* 73(5): 1387-1393.

Deslauriers, R., J. K. Saunders, et al. (1996). Magnetic resonance studies of the effects of cardiovascular surgery on brain metabolism and function. *J Cardiothorac Vasc Anesth* 10(1): 127-137; quiz 137-128.

Djaiani, G., L. Fedorko, et al. (2004). Mild to moderate atheromatous disease of the thoracic aorta and new ischemic brain lesions after conventional coronary artery bypass graft surgery. *Stroke* 35(9): e356-358.

Douglas, J. M., Jr.&S. E. Spaniol (2009). A multimodal approach to the prevention of postoperative stroke in patients undergoing coronary artery bypass surgery. *Am J Surg* 197(5): 587-590.

Glas, K. E., M. Swaminathan, et al. (2008). Guidelines for the performance of a comprehensive intraoperative epiaortic ultrasonographic examination: recommendations of the American Society of Echocardiography and the Society of Cardiovascular Anesthesiologists; endorsed by the Society of Thoracic Surgeons. *Anesth Analg* 106(5): 1376-1384.

Hammon, J. W., Jr., D. A. Stump, et al. (1997). Risk factors and solutions for the development of neurobehavioral changes after coronary artery bypass grafting. *Ann Thorac Surg* 63(6): 1613-1618.

Mahanna, E. P., J. A. Blumenthal, et al. (1996). Defining neuropsychological dysfunction after coronary artery bypass grafting. *Ann Thorac Surg* 61(5): 1342-1347.

Rosenberger, P., S. K. Shernan, et al. (2008). The influence of epiaortic ultrasonography on intraoperative surgical management in 6051 cardiac surgical patients. *Ann Thorac Surg* 85(2): 548-553.

Royse, A.&C. Royse (2006). A standardised Intraoperative ultrasound examination of the aorta and proximal coronary arteries. *Interact CardioVasc and Thorac Surg* 5: 701-704.

Royse, A. G., C. F. Royse, et al. (2000). Reduced neuropsychological dysfunction using epiaortic echocardiography and the exclusive Y graft. *Ann Thorac Surg* 69(5): 1431-1438.

Royse, A. G., C. F. Royse, et al. (1999). Exclusive Y graft operation for multivessel coronary revascularization. *Ann Thorac Surg* 68(5): 1612-1618.

Royse, C., A. Royse, et al. (1998). Assessment of thoracic aortic atheroma by echocardiography: a new classification and estimation of risk of dislodging atheroma during three surgical techniques. *Ann Thorac Cardiovasc Surg* 4(2): 72-77.

Royse, C., A. Royse, et al. (1998). Screening the thoracic aorta for atheroma: a comparison of manual palpation, transesophageal and epiaortic ultrasonography. *Ann Thorac Cardiovasc Surg* 4: 347-350.

Shroyer, A. L., L. P. Coombs, et al. (2003). The Society of Thoracic Surgeons: 30-day operative mortality and morbidity risk models. *Ann Thorac Surg* 75(6): 1856-1864; discussion 1864-1855.

Suvarna, S., A. Smith, et al. (2007). An intraoperative assessment of the ascending aorta: a comparison of digital palpation, transesophageal echocardiography, and epiaortic ultrasonography. *J Cardiothorac Vasc Anesth* 21(6): 805-809.

Sylivris, S., P. Calafiore, et al. (1997). The intraoperative assessment of ascending aortic atheroma: epiaortic imaging is superior to both transesophageal echocardiography and direct palpation. *J Cardiothorac Vasc Anesth* 11(6): 704-707.

Van Zaane, B., N. P. Zuithoff, et al. (2008). Meta-analysis of the diagnostic accuracy of transesophageal echocardiography for assessment of atherosclerosis in the ascending aorta in patients undergoing cardiac surgery. *Acta Anaesthesiol Scand* 52(9): 1179-1187.

Vanninen, R., M. Aikia, et al. (1998). Subclinical cerebral complications after coronary artery bypass grafting: prospective analysis with magnetic resonance imaging, quantitative electroencephalography, and neuropsychological assessment. *Arch Neurol* 55(5): 618-627.

Whitley, W. S.&K. E. Glas (2008). An argument for routine ultrasound screening of the thoracic aorta in the cardiac surgery population. *Semin Cardiothorac Vasc Anesth* 12(4): 290-297.

Yamaguchi, A., H. Adachi, et al. (2009). Efficacy of intraoperative epiaortic ultrasound scanning for preventing stroke after coronary artery bypass surgery. *Ann Thorac Cardiovasc Surg* 15(2): 98-104.

Zamvar, V., D. Williams, et al. (2002). Assessment of neurocognitive impairment after off-pump and on-pump techniques for coronary artery bypass graft surgery: prospective randomised controlled trial. *Bmj* 325(7375): 1268.

Part 2

Echocardiography in Heart Failure

4

Diastolic Heart Failure

Ryotaro Wake*, Junichi Yoshikawa and Minoru Yoshiyama
Osaka City University Graduate School of Medicine
Japan

1. Introduction

The mortality, hospitalization, and prevalence rates of heart failure (HF) are increasing, in spite of decrease in coronary artery and cerebrovascular disease mortality.[1] Importantly, heart failure with normal ejection fraction (HFNEF) currently accounts for more than 50% of all heart failure patients and as the prevalence of HFNEF in the heart failure population rises by 1% a year.[2]

Approximately half of patients with a diagnosis of heart failure have a normal left ventricular (LV) ejection fraction (EF) without valve disease which is defined as diastolic heart failure (DHF), because it is attributed to LV diastolic dysfunction.[3] The prevalence of DHF increase even more dramatically with age more than HF with a reduced EF and is much more common in women than in men at any age. Studies examining prevalence of diastolic heart failure in hospitalized patients or in patients undergoing outpatient diagnostic screening and prospective community based studies have shown that the prevalence of diastolic heart failure approaches 50%.[4-6] Although HF patients with preserved systolic function has a slightly better prognosis than HF patients with abnormal systolic function, there is a fourfold higher mortality risk compared with subjects free of HF.[7]

2. The mechanism of DHF

Heart failure is a clinical syndrome characterized by symptoms and signs of increased tissue water and decreased tissue perfusion. Definition of the mechanisms that cause this clinical syndrome requires measurement of both systolic and diastolic function. When heart failure is accompanied by a predominant or isolated abnormality in diastolic function, this clinical syndrome is called diastolic heart failure. The pathophysiology is attributed to LV diastolic dysfunction, in which LV diastolic chamber size is normal or reduced despite elevated filling pressures resulting in decreased cardiac output. DHF occurs when the ventricular chamber is unable to accept an adequate volume of blood during diastole, because of a decrease in ventricular relaxation and/or an increase in ventricular stiffness,[3] and increased circulating blood volume is present. Hypertension, ischemia, aging and diabetes mellitus are the major risk factor of a decrease in ventricular relaxation and/or an increase in ventricular stiffness. Endocardial biopsies from HF patients without coronary artery

*Corresponding Author

disease (CAD) showed structural and functional differences in cardiomyocytes from patients with diastolic HF compared to cardiomyocytes from patients with abnormal systolic ejection fraction.[8] Myocytes from patients with diastolic HF had increased diameter and higher myofibrillar density and developed greater passive force and had greater calcium sensitivity. Myocardial collagen volume fraction was equally elevated.

2.1 Characteristics of medical examination

Patients with DHF were shown to have similar pathophysiological characteristics, compared with HF patients with a reduced EF including reduced exercise capacity and impaired quality of life. The Framingham criteria for diagnosis of HF is the following. Major criteria are 1) paroxysmal nocturnal dyspnea or orthopnea, 2) jugular venous distention (or central venous pressure is more than 16 mmHg), 3) hearing rale or acute pulmonary edema, 4) cardiomegaly, 5) hepatojuglar reflex, and 6) response to diuretics (weight loss is more than 4.5 kg per 5 days). Minor criteria are 1) ankle edema, 2) nocturnal cough, 3) exertional dyspnea, 4) pleural effusion, 5) vital capacity lower less than two thirds of normal condition, 6) hepatomegaly, and 7) tachycardia (more than 120 beats/minute. With diastolic HF, fourth heart sounds may be present but third heart sounds are seldom present. Chest radiography will show pulmonary congestion during acute exacerbations and for some time following an episode, cardiomegaly will be present in systolic HF but may or may not be present in HF with preserved ejection fraction. When it is difficult with diagnosing HF, it is important to use echocardiography. [9,10]

2.2 The diagnosis of DHF

The diagnosis of heart failure with normal left ventricular (LV) ejection fraction (HFNEF) requires the following conditions to be satisfied: (1) signs or symptoms of heart failure; (2) normal or mildly abnormal systolic LV function; (3) evidence of diastolic LV dysfunction. Normal or mildly abnormal systolic LV function implies both an LVEF > 50% and an LV end-diastolic volume index (LVEDVI) < 97 mL/m^2. Diagnostic evidence of diastolic LV dysfunction can be obtained invasively (LV end-diastolic pressure >16 mmHg or mean pulmonary capillary wedge pressure >12 mmHg) or non-invasively by tissue Doppler (TD) (E/E' >15) with an echocardiography. If TD yields an E/E' ratio suggestive of diastolic LV dysfunction (8 < E/E' < 15), additional non-invasive investigations are required for diagnostic evidence of diastolic LV dysfunction. These can consist of blood flow Doppler of mitral valve or pulmonary veins, echocardiographic measures of LV mass index or left atrial volume index, electrocardiographic evidence of atrial fibrillation, or plasma levels of natriuretic peptides. If plasma BNP is more than 200 pg/mL, diagnostic evidence of diastolic LV dysfunction also requires additional non-invasive investigations (Fig. 1).

LVEDVI: left ventricular end-diastolic volume index, mPCW: mean pulmonary capillary wedge pressure, LVEDP: left ventricular end-diastolic pressure, TD: tissue Doppler, E: early mitral valve flow velocity, E': early TD lengthening velocity, BNP: brain natriuretic peptide, E/A: ratio of early (E) to late (A) mitral valve flow velocity, Dct: deceleration time, LVMI: left ventricular mass index; LAVI: left atrial volume index, Ard: duration of reverse pulmonary vein atrial systole flow, Ad: duration of mitral valve atrial wave flow.

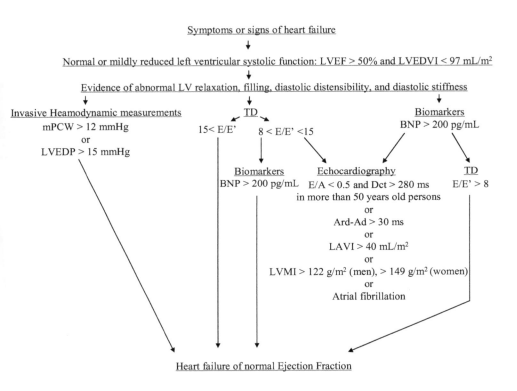

Symptoms or signs of heart failure

Normal or mildly reduced left ventricular systolic function: LVEF > 50% and LVEDVI < 97 mL/m²

Evidence of abnormal LV relaxation, filling, diastolic distensibility, and diastolic stiffness

Invasive Heamodynamic measurements
mPCW > 12 mmHg
or
LVEDP > 15 mmHg

TD
15< E/E'   8 < E/E' <15

Biomarkers
BNP > 200 pg/mL

Biomarkers
BNP > 200 pg/mL

Echocardiography
E/A < 0.5 and Dct > 280 ms
in more than 50 years old persons
or
Ard-Ad > 30 ms
or
LAVI > 40 mL/m²
or
LVMI > 122 g/m² (men), > 149 g/m² (women)
or
Atrial fibrillation

TD
E/E' > 8

Heart failure of normal Ejection Fraction

Fig. 1. How to diagnose HFNEF: Diagnostic flow chart in a patient suspected of HFNEF.

A similar strategy with focus on a high negative predictive value of successive investigations is proposed for the exclusion of HFNEF in patients with breathlessness and no signs of congestion. If a patient with breathlessness and no signs of fluid overload has a BNP of less than 100 pg/mL, any form of heart failure is virtually ruled out because of the high negative predictive value of the natriuretic peptides, and pulmonary disease becomes the most likely cause of breathlessness (Fig. 2). [11,12]

As far as diastolic dysfunctuion, in decompensated patients with advanced systolic heart failure (LVEF ≤ 30%, New York Heart Association class III to IV symptoms), tissue Doppler-derived with E/E' ratio may not be as reliable in predicting intracardiac filling pressures, particularly in those with larger LV volumes, more impaired cardiac indices, and the presence of cardiac resynchronization therapy. [13]

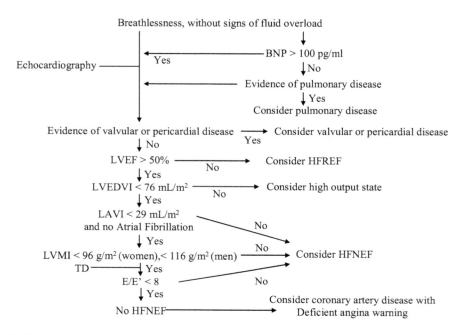

Fig. 2. How to exclude HFNEF: Diagnostic flow chart in a patient presenting with breathlessness and no signs of fluid overload.

2.3 Echocardiography in diastolic heart failure

2.3.1 Doppler echocardiographic assessment of diastolic function and filling pressures

Comprehensive Doppler echocardiography is invaluable in the evaluation of HF patients as the 2.1. characteristics of medical examination section. Assessment of diastolic function begins with the transmitral flow velocity profile. Decreases in the ratio of early to late diastolic filling (E/A), increases in the deceleration time, increases in the isovolumic relaxation time, or increases in tissue Doppler imagings (E/E') indicate impaired relaxation. However, in the presence of impaired relaxation, increases in filling pressure progressively modify the transmitral gradient and mitral inflow pattern. A comprehensive Doppler assessment must be used to determine diastolic function from filling pressures and tissue Doppler imagings. [12] Patients studied at various times during their presentation will display a spectrum of filling patterns, including abnormal relaxation and psuedonormal or restrictive patterns. Such a spectrum has also been reported in patients with HF with a depressed EF and reflects the potent effect of filling pressures and blood pressure and their interaction with underlying diastolic dysfunction on the Doppler patterns. Thus, depending on their level of compensation and their filling pressures and whether they have exertional or rest symptoms, patients with HF preserved EF may display any of the filling patterns.[14]

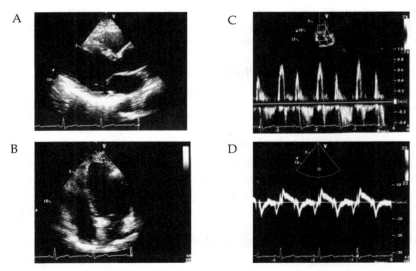

Fig. 3. Normal pattern in LV inflow: Panel A shows long axis view. Panel B shows 4 chamber view. Panel C shows LV inflow. Panel D shows tissue Doppler imaging.

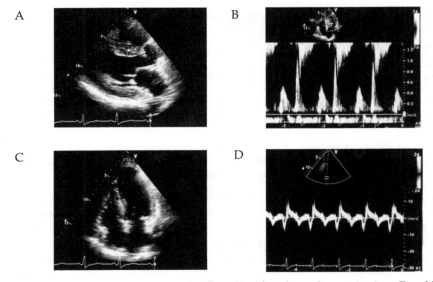

Fig. 4. Abnormal relaxation pattern in LV inflow: Panel A shows long axis view. Panel B shows 4 chamber view. Panel C shows LV inflow. Panel D shows tissue Doppler imaging.

2.3.2 Left ventricle in diastolic heart failure

Most patients with HF preserved EF have normal chamber dimensions, although a small subset may have variable degrees of LV enlargement.

Although HF preserved EF has been thought to occur primarily inpatients with LVH, studies that have carefully quantified LV mass report that echocardiographic criteria for LVH are met in less than 50% of patients. [15-18]

2.3.3 Left atrium in diastolic heart failure

Increases in the left atrial dimension or volume are commonly present in patients with HF preserved EF. [19-21]

2.3.4 Pulmonary hypertension in diastolic heart failure

Just as chronic pulmonary venous hypertension leads to pulmonary arterial hypertension in HF with reduced EF, the same can occur in HF preserved EF, and an elevated tricuspid regurgitant velocity indicative of pulmonary hypertension is extremely common in HF preserved EF.[19, 22]

2.3.5 Other echocardiographic findings in diastolic heart failure

Regional wall motion abnormalities with preserved EF and right ventricular dilatation, either from ischemic disease or secondary to chronic pressure overload from chronic pulmonary venous hypertension, can also be present at echocardiography in patients with HF preserved EF. Additional negative findings at echocardiography include the absence of valvular disease, pericardial tamponade, pericardial constriction, the presence of congenital heart diseases such as atrial septal defect, other more extensive structural abnormalities are important enough to cause the HF symptoms.

2.4 The treatment of DHF

Almost randomized, double-blind studies of therapy for HF are studies of systolic dysfunction. Guidelines for the management of patients with chronic HF have been published by several organizations. The management of patients with DHF is not different from that of HF patients with a reduced EF. They include daily monitoring of weight, attention to patient education, and close medical follow-up. The role of cardiac rehabilitation in patients with DHF has also been explored.[23]

The treatment of diastolic heart failure can be demonstrated the following 3 strategies. First, treatment should target symptom reduction by decreasing pulmonary venous pressure at rest and during exertion. Second, treatment should target the pathological disease that caused the diastolic heart failure. For example, coronary artery disease, hypertensive heart disease and diabetes mellitus provide relatively specific therapeutic targets, such as lowering of blood pressure, induction of hypertrophy regression, blood sugar control and treatment of ischemia by increasing myocardial blood flow and reducing myocardial oxygen demand. Third, treatment should target the underlying mechanisms that are altered by the disease processes.

Diuretics are advised for therapy of diastolic HF in the ACC/AHA Guidelines for Evaluation and Management of Heart Failure. The use of diuretics may improve breathlessness in patients with diastolic HF, because circulating blood volume is a major determinant of ventricular filling pressure. In spite of chronic data are lacking on nitrates, they are effective on the diastolic HF in the acute phase, because of deceasing central blood volume by vasodilating. In spite of chronic data are also lacking on human atrial natriuretic peptides, they are effective on the diastolic HF in the acute phase, because of deceasing central blood volume by natriuretic and vasodilating effect. Digoxin was reported to yield symptomatic improvement and decreased hospitalizations without mortality benefit in the DIG study in patients with DHF.[24]

We treat with angiotensin converting enzyme (ACE) inhibitors, angiotensin receptor blockers (ARBs) and aldosterone antagonists in the chronic systolic heart failure patients, because the rennin-angiotensin- aldosterone system (RAAS) plays the pivotal roles on the left ventricular remodeling in HF patients.[25] Recent studies of HF patients with preserved LV function suggest that ACE inhibitors or ARBs may improve functional class, exercise duration, ejection fraction, diastolic filling and LV hypertrophy. In the large randomized trial of perindopril (an ACE inhibitor) for patients older than 70 years with chronic HF and normal or near-normal EF, event rates were lower than anticipated. Some trends toward benefit, primarily driven by reduction in HF-related hospitalizations, were observed at 1 year (PEP-CHF trial).[26] In the CHARM-Preserved Trial, [27] HF patients with an EF higher than 40% were randomized to candesartan (an angiotensin receptor antagonist) or placebo in addition to standard therapy. Fewer patients in the candesartan group than in the placebo group reached the primary endpoint of cardiovascular death or HF hospitalization, a finding that reached statistical significance only after adjustment for nonsignificant differences in baseline characteristics. Then, irbesartan (an ARB) did not improve the outcomes of DHF patients (I-PRESERVE).[28] Although candesartan and irbesartan are angiotensin receptor blockers, the results of the trials are different. These pleiotropic effects may be different. The trial of aldosterone antagonists for DHF patients is going on in DHF patients (TOPCAT trial). Beta blocker has been shown to improve morbidity with diastolic and systolic HF. [29,30] Although calcium channel antagonists can improve measures of diastolic function during short-term use, definitive data with chronic administration for diastolic HF are not available. Recent reports show statins reduce the number of cardiovascular hospitalizations in patients with systolic heart failure, although they did not reduce the primary outcome which is the composite of death from cardiovascular causes, non fatal myocardial infarction and nonfatal stroke.[31,32] A few trials of statins have shown to improve the mortality in patients with DHF [33]. Further investigations are needed.

3. Conclusions

Heart failure with normal left ventricular ejection fraction (HFNEF) currently accounts for more than 50% of all heart failure patients. The updated strategies for the diagnosis and exclusion of HFNEF are useful not only for individual patient management but also for patient recruitment in future clinical trials exploring therapies for HFNEF.

4. Acknowledgments

The authors thank Dr. Takahiro Shiota, MD (Professor, Cedars-Sinai Heart Institute, Cedars-Sinai Medical Center and UCLA, Los Angels, USA), Dr. Homma Shunichi, MD, FACC (the

Department of Cardiology, Columbia University, USA) and Jae K Oh, MD (Professor of Medicine, Mayo Clinic College of Medicine, Consultant in Cardiovascular Disease, Mayo Clinic, Rochester, Minnesota,USA) for the education of the diastology.

5. References

[1] Braunwald, E. (1997) Shattuck lecture--cardiovascular medicine at the turn of the millennium: triumphs, concerns, and opportunities. N Engl J Med 337 (19), 1360-1369

[2] Owan, T.E. et al. (2006) Trends in prevalence and outcome of heart failure with preserved ejection fraction. N Engl J Med 355 (3), 251-259

[3] Redfield, M.M. (2004) Understanding "diastolic" heart failure. N Engl J Med 350 (19), 1930-1931

[4] Aurigemma, G.P. et al. (2001) Predictive value of systolic and diastolic function for incident congestive heart failure in the elderly: the cardiovascular health study. J Am Coll Cardiol 37 (4), 1042-1048

[5] Gottdiener, J.S. et al. (2000) Predictors of congestive heart failure in the elderly: the Cardiovascular Health Study. J Am Coll Cardiol 35 (6), 1628-1637

[6] Kitzman, D.W. et al. (2001) Importance of heart failure with preserved systolic function in patients > or = 65 years of age. CHS Research Group. Cardiovascular Health Study. Am J Cardiol 87 (4), 413-419

[7] Vasan, R.S. et al. (1999) Congestive heart failure in subjects with normal versus reduced left ventricular ejection fraction: prevalence and mortality in a population-based cohort. J Am Coll Cardiol 33 (7), 1948-1955

[8] van Heerebeek, L. et al. (2006) Myocardial structure and function differ in systolic and diastolic heart failure. Circulation 113 (16), 1966-1973

[9] Prasad, A. et al. (2005) Abnormalities of Doppler measures of diastolic function in the healthy elderly are not related to alterations of left atrial pressure. Circulation 111 (12), 1499-1503

[10] Zile, M.R. and Brutsaert, D.L. (2002) New concepts in diastolic dysfunction and diastolic heart failure: Part I: diagnosis, prognosis, and measurements of diastolic function. Circulation 105 (11), 1387-1393

[11] Paulus, W.J. et al. (2007) How to diagnose diastolic heart failure: a consensus statement on the diagnosis of heart failure with normal left ventricular ejection fraction by the Heart Failure and Echocardiography Associations of the European Society of Cardiology. Eur Heart J 28 (20), 2539-2550

[12] Redfield, M.M. et al. (2003) Burden of systolic and diastolic ventricular dysfunction in the community: appreciating the scope of the heart failure epidemic. JAMA 289 (2), 194-202

[13] Mullens, W. et al. (2009) Tissue Doppler imaging in the estimation of intracardiac filling pressure in decompensated patients with advanced systolic heart failure. Circulation 119 (1), 62-70

[14] Bursi, F. et al. (2006) Systolic and diastolic heart failure in the community. JAMA 296 (18), 2209-2216

[15] Chen, H.H. et al. (2002) Diastolic heart failure in the community: clinical profile, natural history, therapy, and impact of proposed diagnostic criteria. J Card Fail 8 (5), 279-287

[16] Kawaguchi, M. et al. (2003) Combined ventricular systolic and arterial stiffening in patients with heart failure and preserved ejection fraction: implications for systolic and diastolic reserve limitations. Circulation 107 (5), 714-720

[17] Kitzman, D.W. et al. (2002) Pathophysiological characterization of isolated diastolic heart failure in comparison to systolic heart failure. JAMA 288 (17), 2144-2150

[18] Zile, M.R. et al. (2004) Diastolic heart failure--abnormalities in active relaxation and passive stiffness of the left ventricle. N Engl J Med 350 (19), 1953-1959

[19] Lam, C.S. et al. (2009) Pulmonary hypertension in heart failure with preserved ejection fraction: a community-based study. J Am Coll Cardiol 53 (13), 1119-1126

[20] Lam, C.S. et al. (2007) Cardiac structure and ventricular-vascular function in persons with heart failure and preserved ejection fraction from Olmsted County, Minnesota. Circulation 115 (15), 1982-1990

[21] Melenovsky, V. et al. (2007) Cardiovascular features of heart failure with preserved ejection fraction versus nonfailing hypertensive left ventricular hypertrophy in the urban Baltimore community: the role of atrial remodeling/dysfunction. J Am Coll Cardiol 49 (2), 198-207

[22] Kjaergaard, J. et al. (2007) Prognostic importance of pulmonary hypertension in patients with heart failure. Am J Cardiol 99 (8), 1146-1150

[23] Pina, I.L. et al. (2003) Exercise and heart failure: A statement from the American Heart Association Committee on exercise, rehabilitation, and prevention. Circulation 107 (8), 1210-1225

[24] Ahmed, A. et al. (2006) Effects of digoxin on morbidity and mortality in diastolic heart failure: the ancillary digitalis investigation group trial. Circulation 114 (5), 397-403

[25] Schrier, R.W. and Abraham, W.T. (1999) Hormones and hemodynamics in heart failure. N Engl J Med 341 (8), 577-585

[26] Cleland, J.G. et al. (2006) The perindopril in elderly people with chronic heart failure (PEP-CHF) study. Eur Heart J 27 (19), 2338-2345

[27] Yusuf, S. et al. (2003) Effects of candesartan in patients with chronic heart failure and preserved left-ventricular ejection fraction: the CHARM-Preserved Trial. Lancet 362 (9386), 777-781

[28] Massie, B.M. et al. (2008) Irbesartan in patients with heart failure and preserved ejection fraction. N Engl J Med 359 (23), 2456-2467

[29] Flather, M.D. et al. (2005) Randomized trial to determine the effect of nebivolol on mortality and cardiovascular hospital admission in elderly patients with heart failure (SENIORS). Eur Heart J 26 (3), 215-225

[30] Ghio, S. et al. (2006) Effects of nebivolol in elderly heart failure patients with or without systolic left ventricular dysfunction: results of the SENIORS echocardiographic substudy. Eur Heart J 27 (5), 562-568

[31] Khush, K.K. et al. (2007) Effect of high-dose atorvastatin on hospitalizations for heart failure: subgroup analysis of the Treating to New Targets (TNT) study. Circulation 115 (5), 576-583

[32] Kjekshus, J. et al. (2007) Rosuvastatin in older patients with systolic heart failure. N Engl J Med 357 (22), 2248-2261

[33] Fukuta, H. et al. (2005) Statin therapy may be associated with lower mortality in patients with diastolic heart failure: a preliminary report. Circulation 112 (3), 357-363

5

Effects of Eptifibatide on the Microcirculation After Primary Angioplasty in Acute ST-Elevation Myocardial Infarction: A Trans-Thoracic Coronary Artery Doppler Study

Dawod Sharif[1,2], Amal Sharif-Rasslan[2,3] and Uri Rosenschein[1,2]

[1]Cardiology Department, Bnai Zion Medical Center, Haifa
[2]Technion, Israel Institute of Technology, Haifa
[3]Mathematics Departmant,The Academic Arab College, Haifa
Israel

1. Introduction

1.1 Extent of disease

Cardiovascular atherosclerosis is the most common disease in the industrial countries. In the United States of America more than 1 million patients every year are admitted to the coronary care unit with suspected acute myocardial infarction (Yusuf et al, 2004; American Heart Association, 2007). The incidence of acute myocardial infarction in USA is 865000, 565000 of them new infarctions annually. In Europe, the situation is similar to the USA, however in northern countries the incidence is higher than in southern countries (Lopez et al, 2006). In the emerging market economies in Eastern Europe, higher cardiovascular mortality is found. The burden of cardiovascular and coronary heart disease in developing countries is approaching that in developed countries. Thus the problem is a worldwide problem and international joint efforts are needed in order to treat this still prevalent disease.

Mortality of acute myocardial infarction is decreasing steadily. This decrease is related to reduction in the prevalence of disease in some countries, improvement of primary prevention and secondary prevention as well as treatment of the acute event (Hunink et al, 1997; Cooper et al, 2000).

1.2 Contemporary treatment

Primary percutaneous coronary intervention (PCI) is the treatment of choice in acute ST elevation myocardial infarction (Grines et al, 1993; Zijlstra et al, 1993; GUSTO, 1997; De Luca et al, 2004).The objective of primary PCI is to restore myocardial perfusion in the coronary bed distal to the occluded culprit artery. The TIMI classification (Chesebro et al, 1987) and myocardial blush grades (van't Hof, 1998; Gibson et al, 2000; Stone et al, 2002) used to assess epicardial coronary artery flow and myocardial perfusion after primary PCI predict outcome after the procedure. However, the TIMI flow and myocardial blush grades are semi-quantitative, invasive, not easily repeatable, and do not reflect subsequent events and processes at the level of the coronary artery and microcirculation. Thus, even with successful primary PCI and the high rate of patency of the culprit artery, left ventricular functional recovery is limited and not well predicted (Stone et al, 1997; Zijlstra et al, 1997).

1.3 Limitations and problems of contemporary treatment

The main goal of primary PCI is to open the occluded epicardial coronary artery, and thus to re-establish blood flow to the jeopardized myocardium. In order to nourish the myocardium, blood must flow through the epicardial coronary artery segments, resistance vessels, arterioles and capillaries before reaching venules and veins. The epicardial coronary arteries are larger than 400 um, serve as conduit vessels and their diameter is regulated by shear stress and do not contribute significantly to pressure drop. Coronary resistance vessels with diameter between 100 and 400 um are affected myogenically mainly by shear stress and luminal pressure. Resistance coronary vessels with diameter less than 100um are sensitive to local tissue metabolism and directly control perfusion to the low pressure capillary bed nourishing the myocardium. Myocardial capillary density is 3500/mm^2 with inter-capillary distance of 17 um , greater in the subendocardium than in the subepicardium (Canty, 2008).

Microvascular injury is the leading cause for the decreased myocardial perfusion observed in about 80% of patients after successful PCI (Gibson et al, 2000; Stone et al, 1997; Zijlstra et al, 1997; Kondo et al, 1998). Various factors contribute to the limited myocardial perfusion, including micro-emboli, platelets, white blood cells, ischemic necrosis, and reperfusion injury(Chesebro et al, 1987; van't Hof, 1998; Gibson et al, 2000; Stone et al, 2002).

1.4 Detection of dysfunction of the microcirculation

As already mentioned, myocardial blush grade as assessed in the catheterization laboratory evaluates the function of the microcirculation.

Extent of resolution of ST-segment elevation after primary angioplasty is an adequate indicator of the function of the microcirculation and myocardial perfusion.

Measurement of coronary flow velocities using Doppler wire and pressure recordings to assess severity of coronary artery stenoses are invasive procedures in addition to other disadvantages (Iliceto et al 1991; Erbel et al, 1991; Kozakova et al, 1994; Donohue et al, 1993; Miller et al, 1994; Di Carli et al, 1995).

Trans-esophageal echocardiography visualizes only the proximal coronary arteries and Doppler sampling is feasible in less than 70% of patients (Joye et al, 1994; Kern et al 1995; Abizaid et al, 1998).

Recent technologic advances in trans-thoracic echocardiography made Doppler sampling of coronary artery velocities possible (Voci et al, 1998; Caiati et al, 1999; Hildick-Smith et al, 2000; Higashiue et al, 2001; Pizzuto et al, 2001; Takeuchi et al, 2001). Contrast agents may

Effects of Eptifibatide on the Microcirculation After Primary Angioplasty in Acute ST-Elevation Myocardial Infarction:
A Trans-Thoracic Coronary Artery Doppler Study

61

enhance the detection rate of coronary velocities (Abizaid et al, 1998; Caiati et al, 1999), however, an experienced operator is essential.

Sampling of blood velocities in the left anterior descending coronary artery is successful almost in all patients. The advantages of Doppler sampling of coronary artery blood velocities is that it is non-invasive and can be repeated easily in the coronary care unit. As we demonstrated recently using transthoracic Doppler, the function of the microcirculation is dynamic and changes after primary angioplasty (Sharif et al, 2008; 2010). After primary coronary intervention in acute myocardial infraction the microcircirculation may improve or deteriorate. Therefore, transthoracic Doppler sampling of coronary artery velocities is even more important than other methods for the evaluation of the function of coronary microcirculation.

1.5 Possible solution for coronary microvascular dysfunction

After having the epicardial coronary artery treated and well open, according to the mechanisms of microcirculatory dysfunction, platelet micro-emboli and changes in platelet activity may have an impact on myocardial perfusion. Therefore, in the present study we examine the effects adjuvant treatment with glycoprotein 2b3a receptor blockers on the function of the microcirculation after primary angioplasty in the setting of acute anterior ST-elevation myocardial infarction.

2. Methods

Forty five consecutive patients with acute ST elevation anterior myocardial infarction undergoing primary PCI were enrolled in the study. All fulfilled the following criteria: 1) First anterior wall ST segment elevation myocardial infarction (STEMI). 2) Primary PCI within 12 hours of the onset of symptoms. 3) Routine informed consent to perform primary PCI. Anterior STEMI was defined as continuous chest pain for at least 30 minutes and ST elevation of at least 2.0mm in ≥2 contiguous precordial ECG leads. Exclusion criteria included one of the following clinical or angiographic findings: Prior bypass surgery, previous anterior STEMI, significant left main artery disease, failed primary PCI.

2.1 Primary PCI

Primary PCI was performed in standard fashion. All subjects were treated with oral clopidogral (600 mg) and aspirin (300 mg) in the emergency department. Thirty one patients were treated with an intravenous bolus injection of heparin (50-70 U/Kg) to achieve coagulation time of ≥ 250msec, Fourteen patients were treated before angioplasty with intravenous eptifibatide as 2 boluses of 180ug/kg, ten minutes apart, and a maintenance infusion at a rate of 2ug/kg/min for 24 hours, and 500 units heparin/hour. Coronary angiography and primary PCI were performed subsequently. Bare metal stents were deployed by high-pressure implantation techniques. Low magnification angiogram at either the right 30 ° or 90 ° lateral projections with prolonged cine was performed to optimize myocardial blush grade (MBG) documentation at the end of the intervention as previously described (van't Hof et al, 1998). All patients were treated with clopidogrel and aspirin for 12 months after the procedure.

2.2 Echocardiography

All patients had complete Doppler echcardiographic studies, within the first 6 hours after primary PCI, 48 hours later, and 5 days after the intervention.

Siemens, Acuson Sequoia echocardiographic system, California, equipped with 3.5-7MHZ transducers was used. All patients had complete Doppler echcardiographic studies, within the first 6 hours after primary PCI, 48 hours after primary PCI, and 5 days after primary PCI.

In order to obtain LAD flows, the color Doppler Nyquist limit was set at 17 cm/sec or power Doppler modality was applied. Systematic attempt to get LAD-color flow were performed. From low parasternal short axis view, search for diastolic color flow in the anterior interventricular groove followed by clockwise rotation was performed, while form apical foreshortened two chamber views LAD diastolic flow was located in the interventricular groove and the counterclockwise rotation of the transducer was performed. Colour Doppler sampling was easy to achieve, branches could be seen (figure 1) and margins of colour jet well delineated allowing measurement of jet width (figure 2).

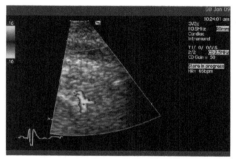

Fig. 1. Colour Doppler of the LAD and diagonal branch

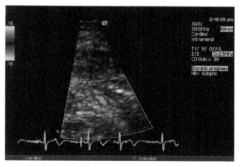

Fig. 2. Colour Doppler of the LAD allowing measurement of jet width

Pulsed-wave Doppler sampling was consistent (figure 3), with dominant diastolic component and clear envelope easy to trace (figure 4) and well demonstrated systolic component (figure 5).

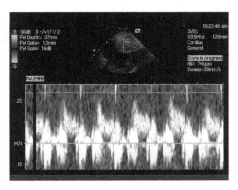

Fig. 3. Consistent pulsed-wave Doppler sampling of LAD blood velocity

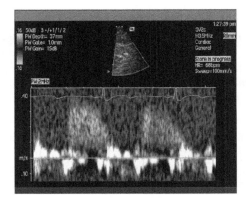

Fig. 4. Pulsed-wave Doppler of LAD blood velocity with dominant, easy to trace diastolic component

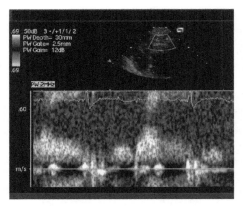

Fig. 5. Pulsed-wave Doppler of LAD blood velocity with prominent systolic flow

2.3 Echocardiographic measurements

Chamber diameters and usual measurements were performed according to recommendations of American Society of Echocardiography. Ejection fraction of LV (LVEF) was measured from biplane apical views.

For the calculation of wall motion score index

$$LV - WMSI = \frac{\sum score\ of\ 16\ segments}{16} \tag{1}$$

assigning a value of 1 for normal LV wall motion, 2 for hypokinesis and 3 for akinesis. Using the same values of wall motion scores, LAD 9 segmental score index was calculated as:

$$LAD - WMSI = \frac{\sum score\ of\ 9\ segments}{9} \tag{2}$$

2.4 Velocity of the LAD and measurements

In order to obtain LAD flows, the color Doppler Nyquist limit was set at 17 cm/sec. From low parasternal short axis view, search for diastolic color flow in the anterior interventricular groove followed by clockwise rotation was performed, while form apical foreshortened two chamber views LAD diastolic flow was located in the interventricular groove and the counterclockwise rotation of the transducer was performed.

Parameters of LAD velocity patterns were averaged from 3 beats, all in sinus rhythm. Diastolic LAD deceleration Time (DDT) was measured as the time from peak diastolic velocity to the intercept of tangent of the velocity envelope with baseline. Pressure half time (P1/2T) (msec) was determined as the time for peak diastolic velocity to decrease to $\frac{1}{\sqrt{2}}$ of its initial value. In addition, search for LAD early systolic flow reversal with early systolic negative velocity (ESFR) was performed.

2.5 LAD Flow measurements

Diameter of the jet of blood velocity through the LAD (D), heart rate (HR) and diastolic time velocity integral (TVI$_{Diastole}$) of the pulsed-wave Doppler were used to calculate blood flow in the LAD according to the following formula (3):

$$Diastolic\ LAD\ Flow = \pi \frac{D^2}{4} \times HR \times TVI_{Daistole} \tag{3}$$

2.6 Angiographic analysis

Coronary angiograms were reviewed by two experienced interventional cardiologists. TIMI (thrombolysis in myocardial infarction) and MBG (myocardial blush grade) were evaluated pre and post- PCI. TIMI-0: no antigrade flow beyond the occlusion; TIMI-1: contrast passes through the occlusion but do not opacify the distality entirely; TIMI-2: contrast passes through the obstruction and opacify the distal coronary bed slower than normal or clears slower than normal; TIMI-3: prompt contrast opacification and clearance of the distal coronary bed (Chesebro et al, 1987). MBG was evaluated as: MBG-0: minimal or no myocardial blush; MBG-1: myocardial staining persists on the next injection; MBG-2: myocardial staining with slow washout and persists markedly at the end of injection; MBG-3: normal myocardial staining and clearance with only mild staining at end of injection (van't Hof, 1998; Gibson et al, 2000; Stone et al, 2002).

2.7 Statistical analysis

Statistical analyses wee conducted using SPSS software version 13. All values were expressed as means and standard deviations. Two-tailed student's-t test was performed to compare changes in DDT and P1/2T, considering $p<0.05$ as statistically significant. Assessment of clinical utility of flow parameters was done by calculating sensitivity, specificity, positive and negative predictive values as well as diagnostic accuracy. Correlation coefficients and their p value were calculated to evaluate the relation of LAD flow parameters with LV systolic function parameters pre-discharge (5 days after PCI).

3. Results

3.1 Angiographic results

Average TIMI and myocardial blush grades (MBG) before angioplasty were not different between patient who were treated with epititifbatide compared to those in whom the medicine was not administrated (table 1). However, TIMI=0, was observed in 33% with eptifibatide compared to 55% in those without. In both groups TIMI and MBG grades improved after the PCI. TIMI grade after the intervention was higher in subjects who were treated with epifibatide, however, MBG was not different.

	TIMI Pre-PPCI	TIMI Post-PPCI	TIMI p-(Pre/Post)	MBG Pre-PPCI	MBG Post-PPCI	MBG p-(Pre/Post)	Diastolic LAD Flow (ml/min)
EPT-Yes	1.07±1.07	2.43±0.5	0.0004	0.71±1.07	1.93±0.73	0.002	49±26
EPT-NO	0.94±1.2	2.28±0.6	$1.3×10^{-9}$	0.52±1.06	2.25±0.9	$6×10^{-9}$	35±17
P (Yes/No)	0.7	0.049		0.57	0.22		0.09

Table 1. Pre and Post PCI, TIMI and MBG and Diastolic LAD Flow

3.2 Feasibility and examples of LAD Doppler velocity sampling

Sampling of LAD blood velocities was possible at all occasions in all the patients. Colour-Doppler jet of blood velocity through the LAD had distinct boarders and measurement of diameters was possible with inter and intra-observer variability of 0.1±0.05mm and 0.15±0.07mm. Inter and intra-observer variability of LAD velocities were 2±0.4 and 1.5±0.2 cm/sec and of time velocity integrals 0.4±0.1 and 0.3±0.1cm, and of pressure half time 10±3 and 8±3 msec In figure 6, an example of a patient with acute anterior STEMI after primary angioplasty and bare metal stent implantation in the LAD. The velocity profile demonstrates prolonged diastolic deceleration time (more than 600msec) and forward systolic flow. In this patient left ventricular systolic function improved and left ventricular ejection fraction at discharge was normal. In figure 7, an example of a patient with unfavorable LAD blood velocity profile after primary angioplasty and bare metal stent implantation in a patient with acute anterior STEMI. Short diastolic deceleration time (less than 600msec) and early systolic flow reversal are demonstrated. In this patient left ventricular ejection fraction was reduced at admission and did not improve later.

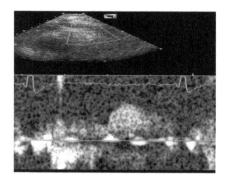

Fig. 6. Favourable LAD blood velocity profile with prolonged diastolic deceleration time and forward systolic flow.

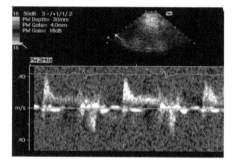

Fig. 7. Unfavourable LAD blood velocity profile with reduced diastolic deceleration time and early systolic flow reversal.

3.3 LAD velocity profiles

Early systolic flow reversal did not occur with eptifibatide while it was noticed in 6 (17%) in those without, p<0.05 (table 2).

	ESFR Early	ESFR 48 Hr.	ESFR 5 Days
EPT-Yes	0	0	0
EPT-No	6	4	2

Table 2. LAD Systolic Flow Reversal

Diastolic deceleration time of LAD flow averaged 629±238 msec in patients treated with eptifibatide and 593±344 msec in those without, p=0.7 (figure 8). Short (<600msec) diastolic deceleration time occurred in 6 (40%) of those treated with eptifibatide, compared to 12 (39%) in those not treated, p=ns (figure 8).

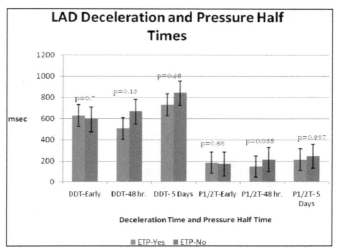

Fig. 8. Histogram of diastolic deceleration time and pressure half time of LAD blood velocity profiles in patients with and those without eptifibatide treatment.

Patients treated with eptifibatide had higher diastolic velocities, 39±11 cm/sec, vs 31±9 cm/sec, p=0.043 and tended to have higher diastolic LAD flows, 49±26 ml/min, vs 35±17 ml/min, p=0.09 (figure 9).

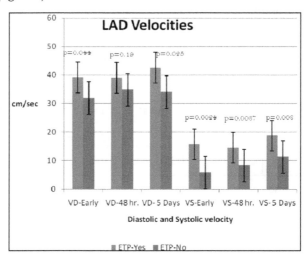

Fig. 9. Histogram of diastolic and systolic velocities of LAD blood velocity profiles in patients with and those without eptifibatide treatment.

3.4 LAD Flow

LAD flow tended to be higher early after primary angioplasty in subjects pre-treated with eptifibatide, however on the following evaluations during mid-hospital stay and pre-discharge diastolic flow in the LAD was similar in both groups.

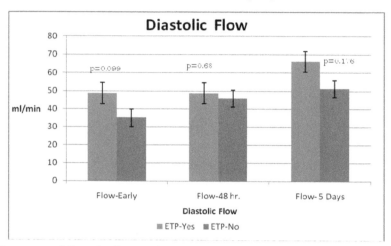

Fig. 10. Histogram of diastolic flow in the LAD in patients with and those without eptifibatide treatment.

3.5 Left ventricular systolic function

LVEF with epifibatide at baseline 37±6.5% was similar to that in those without, 36.7±4.4%, and at discharge, with epifibatide 43.8±8.2% and in those without 45±8.9%, p=ns.

	LVEF (%) Early	LVEF(%) 5 Days	LV-WMSI early	LV-WMSI 5 Days	LAD-WMSI early	LAD-WMSI 5 Days
EPT-Yes	37±6.49	43.8±8.2	1.68±0.17	1.49±0.295	2.15±0.2	1.83±0.43
EPT-NO	36.7±4.4	45±8.9	1.6±0.24	1.39±0.32	2±10.4	1.63±0.55
P (Yes/No)	0.79	0.687	0.296	0.282	0.165	0.258

Table 3. LV Systolic Function

4. Discussion

4.1 Brief summary of results

In this study, per-treatment of patients with acute anterior STEMI undergoing primary coronary angioplasty prevented severe dysfunction of the coronary microcirculation as evidenced by absence of early systolic flow reversal in subjects treated with epitifibatide; however, less severe dysfunction of the microcirculation was not different between the groups since diastolic deceleration times by Doppler, and myocardial blush grades were similar. Moreover, diastolic maximal blood velocities early after PCI were higher in patients treated with eptifibatide but similar later on. Eptfibatide treatment was associated with a tendency of larger diastolic blood flow through the LAD but not later. All these changes with eptifibatide treatment did not affect left ventricular systolic function which was similar in both treatment groups, early after PCI and pre-discharge.

4.2 Applicability of sampling of LAD blood velocities

Transthoracic Doppler sampling of coronary blood velocities is not mentioned or not stressed sufficiently in most textbooks of echocardiography. Thus, the importance of this study is related not only to the treatment of patients with acute STEMI. We found that sampling of LAD blood velocities was possible in all the patients and at all occasions. We believe that sampling of LAD blood velocities should be applied widely and repeated when needed and in all echocardiographic studies. In fact, electrocardiographic recording is performed when patients have chest pain, and in a similar fashion, echocardiography and sampling of coronary blood velocity may be performed in such patients in coronary care units.

4.3 Transthoracic Doppler sampling of LAD blood velocities and other methods

Measurement of coronary flow velocities using Doppler wire and pressure recordings to assess severity of coronary artery and microcirculation are invasive procedures in addition to other disadvantage (Iliceto et al 1991; Erbel et al, 1991; Kozakova et al, 1994; Donohue et al, 1993; Miller et al, 1994; Di Carli et al, 1995). Normal peak diastolic velocities in the present study were similar to those reported previously by invasive Doppler flowires (Ofili et al, 1993).

Trans-esophageal echocardiography visualizes only the proximal coronary arteries and Doppler sampling is feasible in less than 70% of patients (Joye et al, 1994; Kern et al 1995; Abizaid et al, 1998). Recent technologic advances in trans-thoracic echocardiography made Doppler sampling of coronary artery velocities possible (Voci et al, 1998; Caiati et al, 1999; Hildick-Smith et al, 2000; Higashiue et al, 2001; Pizzuto et al, 2001; Takeuchi et al, 2001). Contrast agents may enhance the detection rate of coronary velocities (Abizaid et al, 1998; Caiati et al, 1999), however, with increasing experience of the operator contrast agents are not needed.

4.4 Validity of LAD blood velocities and flow calculations

The range of the value of LAD blood velocities and time velocity integrals (Sharif et al, 2010) is similar to those found through cardiac valves with similar reproducibility and applicability. The diameter of the LAD and of the colour jet of blood flow through the vessel is in the range of diameter of vena contracta of regurgitant jets through cardiac valves. Moreover, LAD-colour jet diameter is similar to that of proximal iso-velocity surfaces of regurgitant jets through the mitral valve, so it can be applied in a similar fashion and squared to calculate areas. Thus if blood velocities, and colour jet diameters of the LAD are similar to those of cardiac valves, then flow calculations should be of the same degree of validity.

4.5 Need for coronary blood velocity sampling in acute STEMI

Restoration of epicardial coronary artery flow by primary PCI in the setting of acute STEMI improves outcome (Shah et al, 2000), however optimization of myocardial tissue perfusion improves the prediction of outcome (van't Hof et al, 1998; Shah et al, 2000; van't Hof et al, 1997; Claeys et al, 1999; The TIMI Study Group, 19985; Gibson et al, 1996; 1999; 2001; de Lemos, 2001; Dörge et al, 2000). Despite these findings, still even with successful primary PCI and the high rate of patency of the culprit artery, left ventricular functional recovery is limited and not well predicted (Stone et al, 1997; Zijlstra et al, 1997).

 Despite the value of myocardial blush grade in the evaluation of myocardial perfusion it is not repeatable because of its invasive nature. Resolution of ST-elevation also correlates with better myocardial perfusion, however it reflects only the stage immediately following the emergency PCI. As we have shown (Sharif et al, 2008) the function of coronary microcirculation is variable and may improve or worsen during the hospital stay after primary coronary angioplasty in patients with acute STEMI. Therefore, Doppler transthorcaic sampling of LAD blood velocities is important in such patients.

4.6 Diastolic deceleration time of LAD blood velocity curve (DDT) and the microcirculation

To understand the relation between DDT and coronary microcirculation, consider normal subjects where the intra-myocardial blood capacitance vessels fill during diastole without significant increase in intramural pressure, therefore the DDT is prolonged. When the capacitance vessels are partially obstructed with miroemboli there is impedance to flow in diastole, therefore the DDT is abbreviated (Kawamoto et al, 1999; Yamamaro et al, 2002). When the blockage of the microcirculation is more severe, the milking of blood in systole cannot proceed to the venules; instead, it is pushed back into the coronary artery and results in early systolic flow reversal (Kawamoto et al, 1999; Yamamaro et al, 2002).

4.7 Mechanisms of dysfunction of coronary microcirculation after primary coronary angioplasty

After primary PCI, dysfunction of the microcirculation may develop as a result of periprocedural microembolization to the distal coronary artery bed. In addition, recently, evidence for the hypothesis that in situ inflammation and thrombosis contributes to dysfunction of the microcirculation after primary PCI was provided (Dörge et al, 2000). Despite the tendency of microemboli to dissolve after they developed during primary PCI, in situ microcirculatory thrombosis may account for worsening of microcirculatory function late after primary PCI. Thus not only early evaluation of the coronary microcirculation is important; in fact the worst coronary microcirculatory status like minimal diastolic deceleration time of LAD blood velocity seems to be even more important.

4.8 The logic and need for intense antiplatelet treatment in acute STEMI

Plaque disruption is considered to be the common substrate of acute coronary syndromes (Boersma et al, 2003). Consequently, the blood is exposed to a significant quantity of thrombogenic materials initiating platelet aggregation and the lumen of the coronary artery become obstructed by a combination of platelets, fibrin and red blood cells. Moreover, as mentioned previously, primary coronary angioplasty in patients with acute STEMI is associated with microembilzation rich with platelets to the distal coronary circulation. Therefore, the administration of rapidly acting powerful antiplatelet agent seems logical. Glycoprotein IIbIIIa receptor blockers fulfil these requirements.

4.9 The evidence of effectiveness of Glycoprotein IIbIIIa receptor blockers in acute STEMI

Thus, Abciximab (Neumann et al, 1998) maintained patency of large coronary arteries, but in addition was associated with higher coronary artery peak blood velocities and better left ventricular wall motion score index and higher left ventricular ejection fraction compared to heparin. Abciximab (de Lemos et al, 2000) was shown to improve both epicardial coronary artery flow and myocardial reperfusion as evidenced by resolution of ST elevation in patients with acute STEMI. Eptifibatide and tirofiban- small molecule Glycoprotein IIbIIIa receptor blockers- in a meta-analysis study were shown to be non-inferior to abciximab in patients with acute STEMI undergoing PPCI (Ottani et al, 2010). Eptifibatide was shown to be equal to abciximab as an adjunct to PPCI in acute STEMI and as effective in causing resolution of ST elevation (Zeymer et al, 2010) and reduced the rate one year mortality and re-infarction (Akerblom et al, 2010). Eptifibatide improved clinical outcome in patients with STEMI undergoing PPCI (Mahmoudi et al, 2011). In our study eptifibatide prevented severe dysfunction of coronary microcirculation after PPCI in acute STEMI which was not translated into better left ventricular systolic function. A larger number of patients may reveal such benefit in recovering left ventricular systolic function.

5. Summary and look to the future

Thus, transthoracic Doppler echocardiography is feasible and provides important information about the function of coronary microcirculation in patients with acute STEMI undergoing PPCI. Treatment with eptifibatide before primary angioplasty, prevented early LAD systolic flow reversal indicative of severe dysfunction of the microcirculation, increased diastolic LAD velocities and flows but did not increase left ventricular systolic function. Understanding mechanisms of dysfunction of the coronary microcirculation and implementation of newer strategies to treat microcirculatory dysfunction with transthoracic Doppler evaluation may improve the treatment of patients with acute STEMI undergoing primary angioplasty.

6. References

Abizaid, A.; Mints, G.S.; Pichard, A.D.;Kent, K.M.; Satler, L.F.; Walsh, C.L.; Popma, J.J. & Leon, M.B. (1998). Clinical, intravscular ultrasound, and quantitaive angiographic determinants of the coronary flow reserve before and after percutaneous transluminal coronary angioplasty. *Am J Cardiol*, Vol, 82, pp. 423-428.

Akerblom, A.; James, S.K.; Koutouzis, M.; Lagerqvist, ; Stenestrand, U.; Svennblad, B. & Oldgren, J. (2010). Eptifibatide is noninferior to abciximab in primary percutaneous coronary intervention: results from the SCAAR (Swedish Coronary Angiography and Angioplasty Registry). *J Am Coll Cardiol*, 3; 56(6), pp. 470-475.

American Heart Association: Heart Disease and Stroke Statistics-2007 Update. *Circulation* 115:69,2007.

Boersma, E.; Mercado, N.; Poldermans, D.; Gardien, M.; Vos, J. & Simoons, M.L. (2003). Acute myocardial infarction. The Lancet, Vol. 361, pp. 847-858.

Caiati, C.; Montaldo, C.; Zedda, N.; Bina, A. & Iliceto, S. (1999). New noninvasive method for coronary flow reserve assessment: contrast-enhanced transthoracic second harmonic echo Doppler. *Circulation*, 99, pp. 771-778.

Canty, J. M. (2008). Atherosclerotic Cardiovascular Disease, In Libby P, Bonow, R.O.; Mann, D.L. & Zipes, D.P. (Eds.): *BRAUNWALD'S Heart Disease- A Textbook of Cardiovascular Medicine*, 8th ed., pp. 1207-1233.

Chesebro, J.H.; Knatteud, G.; Roberts, R.; Borer, J.; Cohen, L.S.; Dalen, J.; Dodge, H.T.; Francis, C.K.; Hillis, D.& Ludbrook, P. (1987). Thrombolysis in myocardial infarction (TIMI) trial phase I: A comparison between intravenous tissue plasminogen activator and streptokinase. *Circulation* , Vol. 76, pp. 142-154.

Claeys, M.J.; Bosmans, J.; Veenstra, L.; Jorens, P.; De Raedt, H. & Vrints, C.J. (1999). Determinants and prognostic implications of persistent ST-segment elevation after primary angioplasty for acute myocardial infacrtion. *Circulation*, Vol. 99, pp. 1972-1979.

Cooper, R.; Culter, J.; Desvigne-Nckens, P.; Fortmann, S.P.; Friedman, L.; Havlik, R.; Hogelin, G.; Marler, J.; McGovern, P.; Morosco, G.; Mosca, L.; Pearson, T.; Stamler, J.; Stryer, D. & Thom, T. (2000). Trends and disparities in coronary heart disease, Stroke, and other cardiovascular disease in the United States: Findings of the national conference on cardiovascular disease prevention. *Circulation*, Vol. 102, No. 25, pp. 3137-3147.

de Lemos,J.A. & Braunwald, E. (2001). ST-segment resolution as a tool for assessing the efficacy of reperfusion therapy. *J Am Coll Cardiol*, Vol. 38, pp. 1283-1294.

De Lemos, J.A.; Elliot, M.; Gibson, C.M.; McCabe, C.H; Giugliano, R.P.; Murphy, S.A.; Coulter, S.A.; Anderson, K.; Scherer, J.; Frey, M.J.; Van Der Wieken, R.; Van De Werf, F. & Braunwald, E. (2000). Abciximab improves both epicardial flow and myocardial reperfusion in ST-elevation myocardial infarction. *Circulation*, Vol. 101, pp. 239-243.

De Luca, G.; van 't Hof, A.W.; de Boer, M.J.; Ottervanger, J.P.; Hoorntje, J.C.; Gosselink, A.T.; Dambrink, J.H.; Zijlstra, F. & Suryapranata, H. (2004). Time to treatment significantly affects the extent of ST-segement resolution and myocardial blush in patients with acute myocardial infarction treated by primary angioplasty. *European Heart Journal*, Vol. 25, pp. 1009-1013.

Di Carli, M.; Czernin, J.; Hoh, C.K.; Gerbaudo, V.H.; Brunken, R.C.; Huang, S.C.; Phelps, M.E. & Schelbert, H.R. (1995). Relation among stenosis severity, myocardial blood flow, and flow reserve in patients with coronary artery disease. *Circulation*, Vol. 91, pp. 1944-1951.

Donohue, T.J.; Kern, M.J.; Aguirre, F.V.; Bach, R.G.; Wolford, T.; Bell, C.A. & Segal, J. (1993). Assessing the hemodynamic significance of coronary artery stenoses: analysis of translesional pressure-flow velocity relations in patients. *J AmColl Cardiol*, Vol. 22, pp. 449-458.

Dörge, H.; Neumann, T.; Behrends, .M; Skyschally, A.; Schulz, R.; Kasper, C.; Erbel, R. & Heusch, G. (2000). Perfusion-contraction mismatch with coronary microvascular obstruction: role of inflammation. *Am J Physiol*, Vol. 279:H2587-1592.

Erbel, R. (1991).Transesophageal echocardiography: new window to coronary arteries and coronary blood flow. *Circulation*, Vol. 83, pp. 339-341.

Gibson, C.M.; Cannon, C.P.; Daley, W.L.; Dodge, J.T.; Alexander, B.; Marble, S.J.; McCabe, C.H.; Raymond, L.; Fortin, T..; Poole, W.K. & Braunwald, E. (1996). TIMI frame count: a quantitative method of assessing coronary artery flow. *Circulation*, Vol. 93, pp. :879-688.

Gibson, C.M.; Cannon, C.P.; Murphy, S.A.; Ryan, K.A.; Mesley, R.; Marble, S.J.; McCabe, C.H.; Van de Werf, F. & Braunwald, E. (2000). Relationship of TIMI Myocardial Perfusion Grade to Mortality After Administration of Thrombolytic Drugs. *Circulation*, Vol. 101, pp. 125-130.

Gibson, C.M.; Murphy, S.A.; Rizzo, M.J.; Ryan, K.A.; Marble, S.J.; McCabe, C.H.; Cannon, C.P.; de Werf, F.V. & Braunwald, E. (1999). Relationship between TIMI frame count and clinical outcomes after thrombolytic administration. *Circulation*, Vol. 99, pp. 1945-1950.

Gibson, M.C.; de Lemos, J.A.; Murphy, S.A.; Susan, J.; Marble, S.J.; McCabe, C.H.; Cannon, C.P.; Antman, E.M. & Braunwald, E. (2001). Combination therapy with abxiximab reduces angiographically evident thrombus in acute myocardial infarction. A TIMI 14 substudy. *Circulation*, Vol. 103, pp. 2550-2554.

Grines, C.L.; Brown, K.F.; Marco, J.; Rothbaum, D.; Stone, G.W.; O'Keefe, J.; Ovelie, P.; Donohue, B.; Chelliah, N.; Timmis, G.C.; Vliestra, R.E.; Strzelecki, M.; Puchrowicz-Ochoki, S. & ONeill, W.W. (1993). A comparison of immediate angioplasty with thrombolytic therapy for acute myocardial infartction: the Primary Angioplasty in Myocardial Infarction Study Group.*N Eng J Med*, Vol. 328, pp. 673-679.

GUSTO IIb investigators. (1997). A clinical trial comparing primary angioplasty with tissue plasminogen activator for acute myocardial infarction. *N Eng J Med*, Vol. 336, pp. 1621-1628.

Higashiue, S.; Watanabe, H.; Yoki, Y.; Takeuchi, K. & Yoshikawa, J. (2001). Simple detection of severe coronary stenosis using transthoracic Doppler echocardiography at rest. *Am J Cariol*, Vol. 87, pp. 1064-1068.

Hildick-Smith, D. & Shapiro, L.M. (2000). Coronary flow reserve improves after aortic valve replacement for aortic stenosis: an adenosine transthoracic-echocardiograhy study, *J Am Coll Cardiol*, Vol. 36, pp. 1889-1896.

Hunink, M.G.; Goldman, L.; Tosteson, A.N.; Mittleman, M.A.; Goldman, PA..; Williams, LW.; Tsevat, J. & Weinstein, M.C. (1997).The recent decline in mortality from coronary heart disease, 1980-1990. The effect of secular trends in risk factors and treatment. JAMA Vol. 277, PP. 535-542.

Iliceto, S.; Marangelli, V.; Memmola, C. & Rizzon, P. (1991). Transesophageal Doppler echocardiography evaluation of coronary blood flow velocity in baseline conditions and during dipyridamole-induced coronary vasodilatation. *Circulation*, Vol. 83, pp. 61-69.

Joye, J.D.; Schulman, D.S.; Lasorda, D.; Farah, T.; Donhue, B.C. & Reichek, N. (1994). Intracoronary Doppler guide wire versus stress single-photon emission computed tomography thallium-201 imaging in assessment of intermediate coronary stensoses. *J Am Coll Cardiol*, Vol. 24, pp. 940-947.

Kawamoto, T.; Yoshida, K.; Akasaka, T.; Hozumi, T.; Takagi, T.; Kaji, S. & Ueda, Y. (1999). Can coronary blood flow velocity pattern after primary percutaneous transluminal coronary angioplasty predict recovery of regional left ventricular function in patients with acute myocardial infarction? *Circulation*, Vol. 100, pp. 339-345.

Kern, M.J.; Donohue, T.J.; Aguirre, F.V.; Bach, R.G.; Caracciolo, E.A.; Wolford, T.; Mechem, C.J.; Flynn, M.S. & Chaitman, B. (1995). Clinical outcome of deferring angioplasty in patients with normal translesional pressure-flow velocity measurements. J Am Coll Cardiol, Vol. 25, pp. 178-187.

Kondo, M.; Nakano, A.; Saito, D. & Shimono, Y. (1998). Assessment of "microvascular no-reflow phenomenon" using technetium-99m macroaggregated albumin scintigraphy in patients with acute myocardial infarction. J Am Coll Cardiol. 1998; 32:898-903.

Kozakova, M.; Palombo, C.; Zanchi, M.; Distante, A.& L'Abbate, A. (1994). Increased sensitivity of flow detection in the left coronary artery by transesophageal echocardiography after intravenous administration of transpulmonary stable echocontrast agent. *J Am Soc Echocardiography*, Vol. 7, pp. 327-336.

Lopez, A.D.; Mathers, C.D.; Ezzati, M.; Jamison, D.T. & Murray, C.J.L. (eds.) (2006). *Global Burden of Disease and Risk Factors*. Oxford, England, Oxford University Press and Washington, DC. The World Bank.

Mahmoudi, M.; Delhaye, C.; Wakabayashi, K.; Torguson, R.; Xue, Z.; Suddath, W.O.; Satler, L.F.; Kent, K.M.; Pichard, A. & Waksman, R. (2011). Integrilin in patients undergoing primary percutaneous coronary intervention for ST-elevation myocardial infarction. J Inter Cardiol, (ahead of print).

Miller, D.D.; Donohue, T.J.; Younis, L.T.; Bach, R.G.; Aguirre, F.V.; Wittry, M.D.; Goodgold, H.M.; Chaitman, B.R. & Kern, M.J. (1994). Correlation of pharmacological 99m-sestamibi myocardial perfusion imaging with poststenotic coronary flow reserve in patients with angiographically intermediate coronary artery stenoses. *Circulation*, Vol. 89, pp. 2150-2160.

Neumann, F.J.; Basini, R.; Schmitt, C.; Alt, E.; Dirschinger, J; Gawaz, M.; Kastrati, A. & Schömig, A.(1998). Effect of Glycoprotein IIb/IIIa receptor blockade on recovery of coronary flow and left ventricular function after the placement of coronary-artery stents in acute myocardial infarction. *Circulation*, Vol 98,pp. 2695-2701.

Ofili, E.O.; Labovitz, A.J.& Kern, M.J. (1993). Coronary flow dynamics in normal and diseased arteries. *Am J Cardiol*, Vol. 71, 3D-9D.

Ottani, F.; La Vecchia, L.; De Vita, M.; Catapano, O.; Tarantino, F.& Galvani, M.(2010). Comparison by meta-analysis of eptifibatide and tirofiban to abciximab in patients with ST-elevation mayocardial infarction treated with primary percutaneous coronary intervention. *Am J Cardiol*, Vol. 15, No. 106(2), pp.167-174.e1.

Pizzuto, F.; Voci, P.; Mariano, E.; Puddo, P.E.; Sardella, G. & Nigri, A.(2001). Assessment of flow velocity reserve by transthoracic Doppler echocardiography and venous adenosine infusion before and after left anterior descending coronary artery stenting. *J Am Coll Cardiol*, Vol. 38, pp. 155-162.

Shah, A.; Wagner, G.S.; Granger, C.B.; O'Connor, C.M.; Green, C.L.; Trollinger, K.M.; Califf, R.M. & Krucoff, M.W. (2000). Prognostic implications of TIMI flow grade in the infarct related artery compared with continuous 12-lead ST-segment resolution analysis: Reexamining the "gold standard" for myocardial reperfusion assessment. *J Am Coll Cardiol*, Vol. 35, pp. 666-672.

Sharif, D; Rofe, G.; Sharif-Rasslan, A.; Goldhammer, E.; Makhul, N.; Shefer, A.; Hassan, A.; Rauchfleish, S. & Rosenschein, U. (2008). Analysis of serial coronary artery flow patterns early after primary angioplasty: new insights into the dynamics of the microcirculation. *Isr Med Assoc J*, June;10(6), pp. 440-444.

Sharif, D.; Sharif-Rasslan, A.; Shahla, C. & Abinader E.G. (2010). Detection of Severe Left Anterior Descending Coronary Artery Stenosis by Transthoracic Evaluation of Resting Coronary Flow Velocity Dynamics. *Heart International*, Vol. 5:e10, pp. 45-48.

Stone, G.W.; Grines, C.L.; Rothbaum, D.; Browne, K.F.; O'Keefe, J.; Overlie, P.A.; Donohue, B.C.; Chelliah, N.; Vlietstra, R.; Catlin, T., & O'Neill, W.W. (1997). For the PAMI Trial Investigators. Analysis of the relative costs and effectiveness of primary angioplasty versus tissue-type plasminogen activator: the Primary Angioplasty in Myocardial Infarction (PAMI) trial. *J Am Coll Cardiol*, Vol.29, pp. 901–907.

Stone, G.W.; Peterson, M.A.; Lansky, A.J.; Dangas, G.; Mehran, R. & Leon, M.B. (2002). Impact of normalized myocardial perfusion after successful angioplasty in acute myocardial infarction, *J Am Coll Cardiol*, Vol. 39, pp. 591-597.

Takeuchi, M; Miyazaki, C.; Yoshitani, H.; Otani, S.; Sakamoto, K. & Yoshikawa J. (2001). Assessment of coronary flow velocity with transthoracic Doppler echocardiography during dodutamine stress echocardiography. *J Am Coll Cariol* Vol. 38, pp. 117-123.

The TIMI Study Group: The Thrombolysis In Myocardial Infarction (TIMI) trial: phase 1 findings. *N Engl J Med* 1985, Vol.312, pp. 932-936.

Van't Hof, A.W.; Leim, A.; de Boer, M.J. & Zijlstra, F. (1997). Clinical value of 12-lead electrocardiogram after successful reperfusion therapy for acute myocardial infarction. *Lancet*, Vol.350, pp. 615-619.

van't Hof, A.W.; Liem, A.; Suryapranata, H.; Hoorntje, J.C.; de Boer, M.J. & Zijlstra, F.(1998). Angiographic assessment of myocardial reperfusion in patients treated with primary angioplasty for acute myocardial infarction: myocardial blush grade. Zwolle Myocardial Infarction Study Group. *Circulation*, Vol. 97: 2302-2306.

Voci, P.; Testa, G.& Plaustro, G.(1998). Imaging of the distal left anterior descending coronary artery by transthoracic color-Doppler echocardiography. *Am J Cardiol*, (12A): 74G-78G.

Yamamuro, A.; Akasaka, T.; Tamita, K.; Yamabe, K.; Katayama, M.; Takagi, T. & Morioka, S. (2002). Coronary flow velocity pattern immediately after percutaneous coronary intervention as a predictor of complications and in-hospital survival after acute myocardial infarction. *Circulation*, Vol.106:3051-3056.

Yusuf, S.; Vaz, M. & Pais, P. (2004). Tackling the challenge of cardiovascular disease burden in developing countries. *Am Heart J*, 1481:1.

Zeymer, U.; Margenet, A.; Haude, M.; et al. (2010). Randomized compaeison of eptifibatide versus abciximab in primary percutaneous coronary intervention in patients with acute ST-segment elevation myocardial infarction: results of the EVA-AMI trail. *J Am Coll Cardiol*, Vol. 3; 56(6), pp. 463-469.

Zijlstra, F.; Beukema, W.P.; van't, H.A.; Liem, A.; Reiffers, S.; Hoorntje, J.C.; Suryapranata, H. & de Boer MJ.(1997). Randomized comparison of primary coronary angioplasty with thrombolytic therapy in low risk patients with acute myocardial infarction. *J Am Coll Cardiol*. Vol.29, pp. 908–912.

Zijlstra, F.; de Boer, M.J.; Hoorntje, J.C; Reiffers, S.; Reiber, J. & Suryapranata, H. (1993). A comparison of immediate angioplasty with intravenous streptokinase in acute myocardial infarction. *N Eng J Med*, Vol.38, pp. 680-684.

6

Phosphodiesterase-5 Inhibitors Improve Left Ventricular Function in Failing Hearts

Fadi N. Salloum and Rakesh C. Kukreja
Virginia Commonwealth University
Medical Center Richmond, Virginia
USA

1. Introduction

Impaired systolic performance and/or diastolic function have long been detrimental consequences of acute myocardial infarction (AMI), which remains a major cause of morbidity and mortality worldwide. Despite considerable therapeutic improvements, left ventricular dysfunction secondary to infarction continues to pose serious health complications, including heart failure (HF), wherein the heart is unable to maintain a cardiac output appropriate for the requirements of the body. Several factors contribute to HF, including adverse ventricular remodeling, progressive hypertrophy and sustained cell death by apoptosis. Therefore, the search for a therapeutic strategy to overcome or mitigate the progression of HF is of paramount importance.

1.1 PDE-5 Inhibitors

Sildenafil citrate (Viagra™) is the first PDE-5 inhibitor approved for treatment of erectile dysfunction. The discovery of this drug in 1989 was the result of extensive research on chemical agents that hold potential promise in the treatment of coronary heart disease. Initial clinical studies on sildenafil in the early 1990s were not promising with respect to its anti-anginal potential. However, a remarkable side effect was reported by a number of volunteers participating in these investigations; sildenafil seemed to enhance penile erections, which soon thereafter became the main focus of further studies. More than 10 million men worldwide have been treated with sildenafil since its market debut in 1998. Sildenafil is highly specific for PDE-5 inhibition with relatively minor cross-reactivity with PDE-6 (Laties & Fraunfelder, 1999). It has a chemical structure similar to cGMP and inhibits PDE-5 by binding to the cGMP-catalytic sites (Corbin & Francis, 2002) thereby allowing the accumulation of cGMP in the erectile tissue. Two additional agents in this class (vardenafil [Levitra™] (Porst et al., 2001) and tadalafil [Cialis™]) have also been developed and approved by the FDA for treatment of erectile dysfunction and recently sildenafil and tadalafil were approved for treatment of pulmonary arterial hypertension (PAH) (Corbin & Francis, 2002). PDE-5 inhibitors are structurally similar to cGMP and therefore compete with cGMP for binding to PDE-5 at the catalytic site (reviewed in Kukreja et al., 2005). Interestingly, PDE expression has been reported to change in pathologic conditions. For instance, in patients with cardiovascular disease or diabetes, nitric oxide (NO) levels are suboptimal due to endothelial dysfunction [damaged NO synthase (NOS)], and recently myocardial PDE-5 expression has been shown to increase in patients with heart failure (Pokreisz et al., 2009). In this regard, targeting PDE-5 is a promising therapeutic approach for treatment of cardiovascular disease and dysfunction.

2. PDE-5 Inhibitors preserve myocardial function following infarction

A number of pioneering investigations from our laboratory have demonstrated that PDE-5 inhibitors attenuate ischemic injury in animal and cell models (Ockaili et al., 2002; Salloum et al., 2003). In animal models, sildenafil and vardenafil exerted an infarct-sparing effect when given before ischemia (Ockaili et al., 2002; Salloum et al., 2003; Salloum et al., 2006) or at the time of reperfusion (Salloum et al., 2007). Furthermore, chronic treatment with sildenafil immediately after permanent occlusion of the left descending coronary artery (LAD) in mice attenuated ischemic cardiomyopathy (Salloum et al., 2008a). These cardioprotective effects are mediated by activation of protein kinase G (PKG), increased expression of endothelial and inducible nitric oxide synthase (eNOS & iNOS), and augmented Bcl-2/Bax ratio. Due to their powerful anti-ischemic effects, PDE-5 inhibitors became promising candidates for the preservation of cardiac function following AMI. In fact, several studies demonstrated that PDE-5 inhibition preserved left ventricular (LV) function in failing hearts as discussed in the following sections.

2.1 Sildenafil attenuates left ventricular dysfunction in ischemic heart failure

Salloum et al. showed that chronic treatment with sildenafil preserves cardiomyocytes post AMI through reduction of myocardial necrosis, apoptosis and hypertrophy thereby limiting the progression of HF (Salloum et al., 2008a). This study used a murine model of post-MI remodeling by permanent ligation of the left coronary artery. The experimental protocol is illustrated in Figure 1. LV function was assessed at 7 and 28 days post MI. Cardiac function

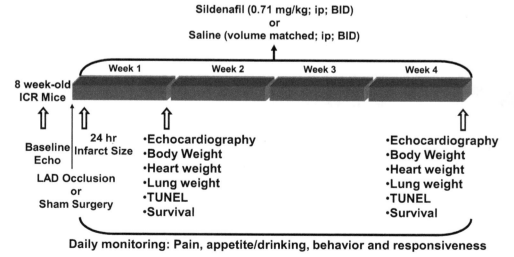

Fig. 1. Experimental protocol illustrating various parameters studied at different time points

was evaluated by echocardiography using the Vevo770™ imaging system (VisualSonics, Inc., Toronto, Canada). A 30-MHz probe was utilized to obtain two-dimensional, M-mode and Doppler imaging from parasternal short-axis view at the level of the papillary muscles and the apical four-chamber view (Schiller et al., 1989). M-mode images of the LV were obtained and systolic and diastolic wall thickness (anterior and posterior) and LV end-systolic and end-diastolic diameters (LVESD and LVEDD, respectively) were measured.

Figure 2 is representative of M-mode images from mice on day 28 post MI. The hearts from sham and sildenafil-treated mice exhibited a smaller LV cavity and thicker infarct wall compared to the saline-treated mice. Increase in LVEDD, LVESD and a decrease in anterior wall diastolic thickness (AWDT), anterior wall systolic thickness (AWST) and fractional shortening (FS) in saline- and sildenafil-treated mice (vs. baseline and sham) were observed on day 7 and 28.

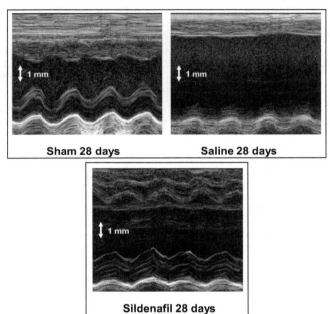

Fig. 2. M-mode images from mouse LV treated with sildenafil or vehicle 28 days after MI

Sildenafil-treated mice had smaller LVEDD, LVESD, greater FS, and lower Tei index (reflecting better myocardial performance) on day 7 and 28 as compared to saline-treated group ($P<0.05$, Figure 3). Sildenafil-treated animals also had a shorter isovolumetric relaxation time (reflective of lower LV end-diastolic pressure) 28 days after AMI when compared to saline-treated animals (11±3 vs. 27±7 ms, respectively, $P=0.03$), which was not different from sham operated animals (10±3, $P=NS$). AWDT and AWST were also greater in sildenafil-treated animals (vs. saline-treated animals, $P<0.05$) on day 7 and 28 post MI showing a protective effect in the peri-infarct region, while no differences in PWDT and PWST were seen. Aneurysmatic dilatation of the anterior wall and apex was observed on day 28 in 90% of saline-treated mice and 62% of sildenafil treated animals ($P>0.05$).

Moreover, the number of aneurysmatic segments [based on a 16-segment map (Schiller et al., 1989)] was 2.9 in saline-treated animals vs. 1.1 in sildenafil-treated animals (P<0.05).

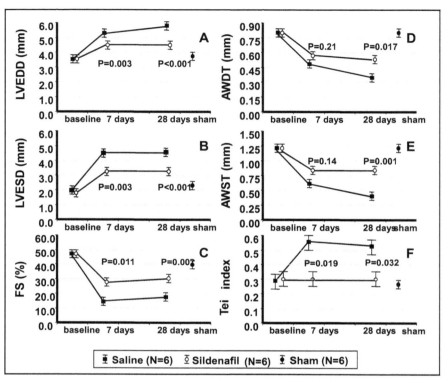

Fig. 3. Echocardiography results of LV function at 28 days post-MI in sildenafil- and saline-treated mice

2.2 Tadalafil preserves left ventricular function following MI through PKG-dependent generation of hydrogen sulfide

We also studied the effect of a longer acting PDE-5 inhibitor, tadalafil, on cardiac function in an acute model of myocardial infarction (Salloum et al., 2009). After baseline transthoracic echocardiography, adult male mice were injected i.p. with vehicle (10% DMSO) or tadalafil (1 mg/kg) with or without KT5823 (KT, PKG blocker, 1 mg/kg) or dl-propargylglycine [PAG, Cystathionine-γ-lyase (CSE, H2S-producing enzyme) blocker; 50 mg/kg] 1 h prior to coronary artery ligation for 30 min and reperfusion for 24 h, whereas C57BL-wild type and CSE-knockout mice were treated with either vehicle or tadalafil. After reperfusion, repeat echocardiography was performed. Similar to sildenafil, tadalafil preserved cardiac performance following MI as compared to vehicle. In this study, since ischemia was limited to 30 minutes, none of the groups presented with significant LV dilatation at 24 h post infarction, however, tadalafil preserved fractional shortening (FS: 31±1.5%) compared to control (FS: 22±4.8%, P<0.05, Figure 4). Baseline FS was 44±1.7%. KT and PAG abrogated the preservation of LV function with tadalafil by a decline in FS to 17±1% and 23±3%, respectively.

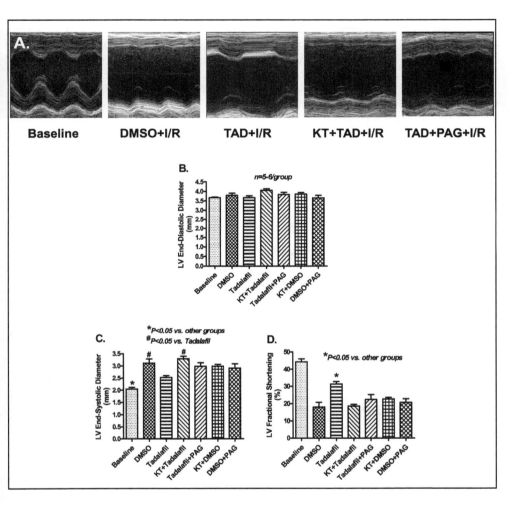

Fig. 4. Tadalafil preserves LV function at 24 hours following MI through PKG and H₂S signaling

2.3 Sildenafil treatment 3 days following MI mitigates the progression of heart failure

In the previous studies, PDE-5 inhibitors were administered either shortly prior to or immediately after infarction. This raises the question whether the preservation of cardiac function observed was a true phenomenon, or it was simply secondary to the anti-infarct effect of these drugs. Specially, little is known about the effects of PDE-5 inhibition on limiting adverse remodeling independent of its ability to modulate infarct size. This concept is clinically relevant, particularly in patients with advanced ischemic HF, because necrosis has a negligible role in a post-infarct setting (Anversa et al., 1993). To address this question, we administered sildenafil 3 days following MI (Chau et al., 2011). Specifically, we sought to determine if sildenafil treatment following LV dysfunction, defined as FS less than 25% at day 3 post-MI, could prevent the progression of HF in a permanent LAD occlusion model. At 3 days post MI, mice receiving sildenafil or saline (control) treatment had similar FS (18±1% and 19±1%, respectively, P>0.05) as compared to baseline value of 47±1%. At days 7 and 28 post-MI, sildenafil-treated group had a significantly higher FS than saline-treated mice (P<0.05). Both LVEDD and LVESD were increased in saline-treated mice as compared to sildenafil-treated mice (P<0.05), indicating more dilatation. Moreover, AWDT was greater in sildenafil-treated animals versus saline-treated animals (P<0.05) on day 28 post-MI. Fractional shortening of sham-operated mice was 43±1.0% at 28 days post left thoracotomy. An increase in LVEDD from a baseline value of 3.5±0.1 mm and a decrease in FS in saline- and sildenafil-treated mice as compared to baseline and sham-operated mice (P<0.05) was observed on days 3 and 28, as shown in figure 5.

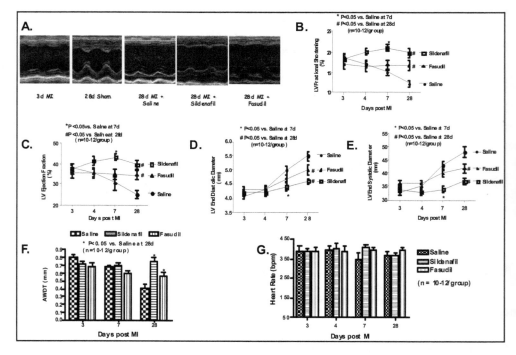

Fig. 5. Late sildenafil treatment preserves LV function and attenuates the progression of ischemic heart failure

2.4 Sildenafil preserves LV function in infant rabbits

Although we previously showed that PDE-5 inhibitors induce powerful preconditioning-like protective effects in the ischemic heart, it is not known whether sildenafil exerts similar protective effects against ischemia/reperfusion injury in the infant rabbit hearts as well. In this study, we used the model of coronary artery occlusion and reperfusion in infant rabbits (Bremer et al., 2005), which is similar to our previously described adult rabbit model of myocardial infarction. The benefits of this work are immense since this model may be applicable in pediatrics, and especially in pediatric cardiovascular surgery where there may be periods of ischemia/reperfusion injury. Also, we used two-dimensional (2D) and Doppler trans-esophageal echocardiography (TEE) for the estimation of LV cardiac output (LVCO) and aortic velocity time integral (VTI) in this model. A 10-Fr AcuNav diagnostic ultrasound probe (Acuson Corp., Siemens, Iselin, NJ) was inserted into the esophagus, at baseline, after the 30 min period of ischemia, and after 3 h of reperfusion in both the control and sildenafil groups. Standardized 2D imaging in a long axis view of the LV to show LV inflow across the mitral valve and LV outflow tract (LVOT) was obtained. Aortic flow Doppler across the aortic valve was performed in a long axis view of the LV and LVOT to obtain LVCO. The standard equation: mean velocity (cm/s) × flow area (cm2) × 60 (s/min), where mean velocity (cm/s) = VTI (in cm/beat) ÷ RR interval (s/beat), was used to obtain LVCO, expressed in milliliters per minute. Laminar Doppler flow across the aortic valve confirmed the absence of aortic stenosis. Color Doppler assessment was made of both the aortic and mitral valves again in the long axis view at baseline, after the ischemic period, and after 3 h of reperfusion for the presence or absence of mitral or aortic regurgitation. Subjective functional assessment was also made after ischemia and reperfusion to demonstrate at least left ventricular apical diminished contractility to confirm infarction. In this study, we showed that both the control and sildenafil-treated groups had comparable LVCO and aortic VTI at baseline. The controls had a decline in LVCO and aortic VTI immediately after the 30-min period of ischemia (28% and 27% lower than baseline values, respectively, $p < 0.05$), whereas the LVCO and aortic VTI increased in the sildenafil group after ischemia (43% and 45% higher than baseline values, respectively, n = 6 per group, $p < 0.05$). Both groups, however, had significant decline in LVCO after 3 h of reperfusion (54% of baseline in the sildenafil group, $p < 0.05$, and 62% of baseline in the control group, $p < 0.05$), and were not statistically significantly different from each other (n = 4–6 per group). Both groups demonstrated a decrease in aortic VTI after 3 h of reperfusion. However, this decline was only statistically significant in the control group compared with baseline values. None of the rabbits had aortic stenosis or developed aortic regurgitation for the duration of the study. Moreover, both the control and sildenafil groups demonstrated a comparable amount of mitral regurgitation (no more than mild) after ischemia/reperfusion, and none of the rabbits had baseline mitral regurgitation.

2.5 Sildenafil and vardenafil preserve LV function in female mice

Since the impact of PDE-5 inhibitors on the female cardiovascular system following ischemia remains unknown, we interrogated the effect of sildenafil and vardenafil on ischemia/reperfusion injury in female mice. In this study, adult female mice were pretreated (ip, bid) with sildenafil (0.7 mg/kg), vardenafil (0.14 mg/kg) or saline one hour before left coronary artery ligation for 30 minutes and reperfusion for 24 hours (Salloum et al., 2008b). Cardiac function, evaluated using echocardiography, showed that LV end-diastolic and end-systolic diameters increased 7 days post myocardial infarction with saline

(3.5±0.1 mm and 2.4±0.2 mm, respectively). In contrast, no dilatation was detected in sildenafil (3.0±0. mm and 1.4±0.1 mm, respectively) and vardenafil (2.9±0.3 mm and 1.4±0.2 mm, respectively) groups. Fractional shortening decreased at 7 days post infarction with saline (30±4%; P<0.05), but was preserved with sildenafil (52±2%) and vardenafil (53±5%). These data clearly suggest that PDE-5 inhibitors induce powerful cardioprotection in female mice as well. For this reason, PDE-5 inhibition may be a novel therapeutic strategy against ischemia/reperfusion injury in women with coronary artery disease.

3. PDE-5 Inhibitors protect against doxorubicin-induced cardiac dysfunction

A number of pioneering investigations from our laboratory have demonstrated that PDE-5 inhibitors attenuate doxorubicin-induced cardiomyopathy in animal and cell models (Koka et al., 2010; Das et al., 2010). In a recent study, we tested whether sildenafil potentiates the antitumor efficacy of doxorubicin in prostate cancer. Our results show that doxorubicin and sildenafil induce a potent antitumor effect in prostate cancer while simultaneously providing a cardioprotective effect. This study was an elegant sequel to our previous work demonstrating that sildenafil attenuated doxorubicin-induced cardiomyopathy in mice (Fisher et al., 2005). In that study, we showed that treatment with sildenafil attenuates the decline in LV developed pressure caused by doxorubicin treatment. An important question, however, was whether sildenafil interferes with the anti-tumor effect of doxorubicin. Our recent study showed that sildenafil ameliorates doxorubicin-induced cardiac dysfunction without interfering with its chemotherapeutic benefits (Das et al., 2010). Cardiac function in nude mice with tumor xenografts was monitored by Doppler echocardiography using the Vevo770 imaging system (VisualSonics, Toronto, Canada) as previously reported (Salloum et al., 2008a). A slight increase in LVEDD and LVESD were observed with doxorubicin. LVFS and LVEF declined in doxorubicin-treated mice. Sildenafil co-treatment with doxorubicin improved LVFS and LVEF compared with the doxorubicin-treated group (P < 0.05). No differences in heart rate were observed between control, doxorubicin, and doxorubicin and sildenafil groups. Sildenafil-treated animals showed lower heart rates compared with other groups (P < 0.01; n = 8). These data suggest that changes in LVFS or LVEF were independent of heart rate.

In a separate study, tadalafil improved left ventricular function and prevented cardiomyocyte apoptosis in doxorubicin-induced cardiomyopathy through mechanisms involving upregulation of cGMP, PKG activity, and MnSOD level without interfering with the chemotherapeutic benefits of doxorubicin (Koka et al., 2010). In these studies, adult male CF-1 mice were randomized to receive saline (0.2 ml i.p.), doxorubicin (15 mg/kg i.p.), or doxorubicin + tadalafil (4 mg/kg p.o. daily) for 9 days starting 3 days before doxorubicin treatment. We chose to use a single dose of doxorubicin at 15 mg/kg i.p., which has been reported to be cardiotoxic. LV function was significantly impaired 5 days after doxorubicin treatment. However, mice treated with doxorubicin + tadalafil showed preserved fractional shortening and ejection fraction compared with those treated with doxorubicin as shown in Figure 6 (n = 6, p < 0.05). In addition, the LV systolic pressure decreased 36%, +dp/dtmax decreased 63%, −dp/dtmax decreased 57%, and heart rate decreased 30% as compared with the controls (P < 0.05). In contrast, mice treated with doxorubicin + tadalafil showed improved LV function (i.e., LV systolic pressure, 33%; +dp/dtmax, 35%; −dp/dtmax, 46%, and heart rate, 27%) as compared with the group treated with doxorubicin alone (n = 6, p < 0.05).

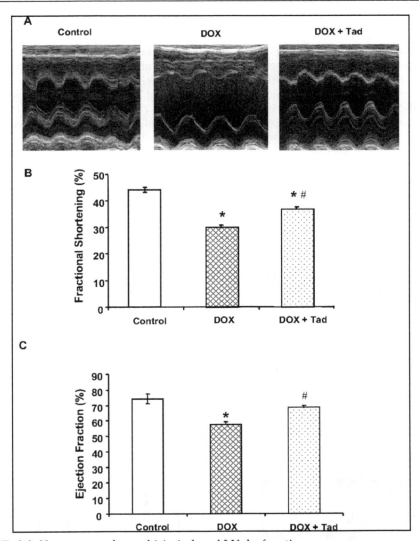

Fig. 6. Tadalafil attenuates doxorubicin-induced LV dysfunction

4. PDE-5 inhibitors protect against hypertrophy-induced cardiac dysfunction

Sustained pressure overload leads to cellular and molecular changes that are initially activated as compensatory mechanisms but later become maladaptive and contribute to progressive cardiac dysfunction and heart failure. This response involves a combination of complex signaling and transcription pathways that induce hypertrophic remodeling (Frey & Olson, 2003; Frey et al., 2004). The heart appears to have an intrinsic signaling system coupled to cGMP that can inhibit myocardial proliferative responses. Several studies using approaches that involve enhanced cGMP synthesis or prevention of its degradation have been shown to blunt hypertrophy despite sustained pressure overload or neurohormonal stress. Interestingly, although cGMP synthesis is often increased by chronic exposure to such stresses, this increase appears to be ineffective to impede hypertrophy and remodeling progression, likely due to increase in PDE-5 expression and activity that accompany such stressors. For this reason, the use of PDE-5 inhibitors to reduce the catabolism may augment cGMP-dependent antihypertrophic effects. In the study by Takimoto et al., the authors show that PDE-5 inhibition with sildenafil prevents cardiac chamber, cellular and molecular remodeling induced by pressure overload (Takimoto et al., 2005). They next tested a more clinically relevant question of whether inhibition of PDE-5 can reverse pre-existing hypertrophy. Mice were exposed to transverse aortic constriction for 7–10 days, which increased heart mass by 63% (P < 0.005) without chamber dilatation. After hypertrophy was established, these mice were divided into 2 groups that received either sildenafil or vehicle for an additional 2 weeks. Cardiomyocyte hypertrophy and interstitial fibrosis were observed in mice exposed to 1 week of transverse aortic constriction, and both reversed to baseline with sildenafil treatment. Serial echocardiography also showed a gradual decline in LV mass and wall thickness, with preservation of systolic ejection in sildenafil-treated mice (Figure 7).

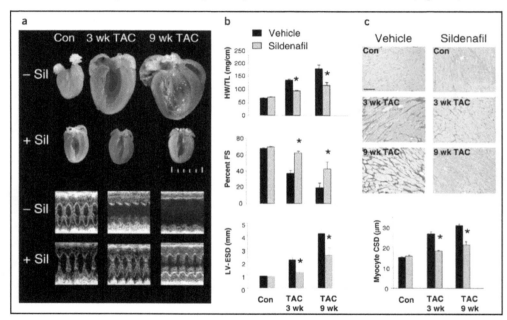

Fig. 7. Sildenafil attenuates and reverses hypertrophy-induced cardiac dysfunction

Another study by Nagayama et al. showed that delayed sildenafil treatment suppresses progressive cardiac dilatation, dysfunction, fibrosis, and hypertrophy in hearts subjected to sustained pressure-overload (Nagayama et al., 2009). In this study, following 3-week transverse aortic constriction, hearts had a +135% increase in LV mass, chamber end-systolic (+91%) and end-diastolic (+10%) dimensions, and reduced fractional shortening (−42%). Subsequent treatment with sildenafil fully arrested progressive remodeling, whereas control hearts further dilated and hypertrophied after 9-week transverse aortic constriction. Postmortem analysis confirmed that both heart and lung weights, normalized to tibia length, were lower with sildenafil treatment. Moreover, cardiomyocyte cross-sectional dimension and interstitial and perivascular fibrosis was also reduced in sildenafil-treated myocardium.

5. PDE-5 inhibitors reverse cardiac dysfunction in Duchenne muscular dystrophy

Duchenne muscular dystrophy (DMD) is a degenerative, muscle-wasting disease caused by mutations in the dystrophin gene. The total loss of dystrophin mainly affects skeletal muscle and results in impaired respiratory function, primarily in older boys (Finsterer & Stöllberger, 2003; Adamo, 2010). Due to remarkable improvement of noninvasive respiratory support in the recent past, the lifespan of patients with DMD has increased. Unfortunately, this was also associated with an increase in the incidence of complications and eventual mortality from cardiomyopathy (McNally, 2008). Cardiomyopathy is a delayed symptom of the disease that usually develops by the second decade of life, with more than 90% of patients presenting clinical symptoms by 18 y of age (Finsterer & Stöllberger, 2003). Loss of cardiac dystrophin eventually leads to dilated cardiomyopathy, which manifests as congestive heart failure in at least 20% of patients (Finsterer & Stöllberger, 2003). Current treatment options for heart failure associated with DMD include angiotensin converting enzyme inhibitors and β-blockers. Despite the moderate benefits provided by these medications in patients with systolic heart failure, similar advantages have not been observed in dystrophic patients with features of systolic and diastolic dysfunction (Bushby, 2003). These findings highlight the need for treatments that slow the development of cardiomyopathy in DMD and improve cardiac function in older patients with established cardiomyopathy.

It has been shown that stimulation of cGMP synthesis by overexpression of cardiac-specific neuronal (n)NOS reduces impulse-conduction defects in dystrophin-deficient (mdx) mice (Wehling-Henricks et al., 2005; Wehling et al., 2001). Similarly, increased particulate guanylyl cyclase activity in young mdx mice has also been shown to decrease susceptibility to cardiac damage during sympathetic stress (Khairallah et al., 2008). These findings clearly implicate reduced NO-cGMP signaling as a key contributor to myocardial pathogenesis in patients with DMD. Therefore, it is plausible that restoration of NO signaling, particularly by preservation of cGMP, may provide therapeutic benefit to dystrophic hearts. In a recent study, Adamo et al. tested whether chronic inhibition of PDE-5 with sildenafil would reverse cardiac dysfunction in the mdx mouse model of DMD (Adamo et al., 2010)

Chronic sildenafil treatment prevented LV functional deficits in aging mdx mice. Furthermore, late sildenafil treatment, i.e. after developing cardiomyopathy, reversed the established symptoms.

Conventional echocardiography and tissue Doppler analysis were used to monitor the development of LV dysfunction in aging mdx mice. Both the myocardial performance index (MPI) and ratios of early diastolic velocity (Ea) to peak velocity with atrial contraction (Aa) were calculated. MPI is a sensitive measure of left ventricular systolic and diastolic performance, whereas the Ea/Aa largely reflects diastolic function. The majority of patients with DMD exhibit diastolic dysfunction and impaired myocardial performance, which can be identified by increased MPI (Bahler et al., 2005). This dysfunction usually precedes the onset of systolic heart failure and dilated cardiomyopathy (Markham et al., 2006). Mdx mice show these same echocardiographic abnormalities (Jearawiriyapaisarn et al., 2010; Townsend et al., 2007).

Three different sildenafil treatment regimens were used: 1- long-term chronic sildenafil treatment starting at 1 month of age, 2- long-term treatment starting at 12 months with echocardiographic measurements taken 3 months later to assess whether established dysfunction could be reversed, and 3- a similar treatment starting at 12 months, but with multiple measurements to determine the time course of the reversal. The results showed impaired LV performance in mdx mice (increased MPI) by 11 to 13 months of age compared with treated and untreated WT controls. As mice approached 15 months of age, mdx mice continued to demonstrate impaired LV function whereas WT control mice began to show a slight age-related decline in cardiac performance. Although sildenafil did not have an effect on cardiac performance in WT mice, mdx mice that received chronic sildenafil treatment starting at 1 month of age retained a relatively normal MPI with age, indicating that sildenafil attenuated the cardiomyopathy in mdx mice. Furthermore, late sildenafil treatment following well-established cardiomyopathy at 12 months of age completely reversed LV dysfunction by age 15 months, as evidenced by normal MPI at that time point. Taken together, these results demonstrate that chronic treatment with sildenafil mitigates the progression of LV dysfunction and late treatment also reverses established LV dysfunction in mdx mice (Figure 8).

In order to better understand the underlying cause for the improvement in the MPI by sildenafil, which could be a result of effects on systolic or diastolic function, the authors measured the Ea/Aa using tissue Doppler imaging to more directly evaluate diastolic function in mdx mice. This parameter largely reflects the diastolic (chamber relaxation and filling) capacity of the LV. As shown in Figure 8B, diastolic dysfunction (indicated by Ea/Aa <1) was observed in mdx mice as early as 8 months of age. Moreover, chronic sildenafil treatment reduced the progression of diastolic dysfunction in mdx mice through 15 months of age. Even when sildenafil treatment was initiated after LV dysfunction was established at 12 months of age, it markedly reversed the diastolic dysfunction within 3 months. Based on this result, the authors suggest that diastolic dysfunction is a major component of the impaired MPI observed in 11- to 13-month-old mdx mice.

Cardiac remodeling after injury can result in hypertrophy, increased fibrosis and systolic dysfunction of the heart. However, cardiomyopathy in mdx mice is characterized by slow, progressive cell death, followed by compensatory hypertrophy of the surviving cardiomyocytes. In order to study the impact of sildenafil on cardiac dimensions and remodeling, the authors used M-mode echocardiography to determine LV dimensions in conscious mdx mice. By 12 months of age, the LV wall thickness of mdx mice was increased and the LV mass index (LVMI) was larger compared with sildenafil-treated mdx mice. Taken together, the anti-hypertrophic effect of sildenafil, coupled with the prevention of diastolic dysfunction, suggest that sildenafil may also have protective effects on some aspects of cardiac remodeling. However, the authors did not find any difference in the FS of 12-month-old, conscious mdx mice compared with WT controls or sildenafil-treated mdx mice, nor did they observe any effect on heart rate. This indicates a lack of major systolic dysfunction in these animals up to 12 month of age. Although systolic dysfunction may develop later in life, it appears that diastolic dysfunction plays a more prominent role in the cardiomyopathy seen in the mdx mice used in this study.Overall, the findings of this study suggest that PDE-5 inhibitors may be an effective treatment for DMD-associated cardiomyopathy at early and late stages of the disease.

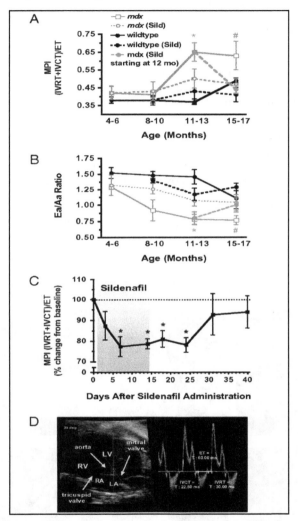

Fig. 8. Sildenafil reverses cardiac dysfunction in the mdx model of Duchenne Muscular Dystrophy

6. Clinical use of PDE-5 inhibitors in patients with heart failure

Following years of basic research examining the cardioprotective effects of PDE-5 inhibitors against ischemia, a recent study by Guazzi et al. demonstrated that sildenafil improves LV diastolic function, cardiac geometry, and clinical status in patients with stable systolic heart failure (Guazzi et al., 2011). The study primarily focused on the effects of chronic PDE-5 inhibition on LV diastolic function and cardiac chamber remodeling, providing the first human evidence that PDE-5 inhibition can be beneficial for improving the diastolic and structural properties of the failing LV. Transthoracic echocardiography was performed using IE33, Philips ultrasound machine, equipped with a software for tissue Doppler (TD), using a 2.5- to 5.0-MHz probe (S5). Standard M-mode, 2D, and Doppler blood flow measurements were performed according to the current American Society of Echocardiography Guidelines (Quiñones et al., 2002). Chamber dimensions were obtained using standard procedures including left atrial volume index (LAVI) and LV mass index (LVMI) (Devereux & Reichek, 1977). Septal and posterior wall thickness, LA, and LV end-systolic and end-diastolic dimensions were obtained from the parasternal long-axis view. LVEF, end-diastolic volume index (LVEDVI), and end-systolic volume index were evaluated with the Simpson method.

Interestingly, E/E', a variable repeatedly found related to LV filling pressures in a variety of left-sided cardiac disorders (Lester et al., 2008), significantly decreased at 6 months and 1 year of active treatment (Figure 9). Additional study findings that support the hypothesis that PDE-5 inhibition may represent a novel and viable therapeutic strategy for improving LV relaxation were the significant shortening in both lateral and septal T E-E', a Doppler-derived index of LV relaxation performance validated against invasively measured negative dP/dT22, and the reverse remodeling effect on LV mass. Moreover, over 12 months, LAVI, LVEDV, and LVMI were unchanged in the placebo group and decreased in the active treatment group, which suggests reverse remodeling with sildenafil involving both the ventricle and the atrium. Over the same time period in the sildenafil group, there was a progressive increase in mean LVEF, from 29.5% at baseline to 34.9% and 36.3% at 6 and 12 months, respectively (P<0.01). Changes observed with sildenafil were significantly different

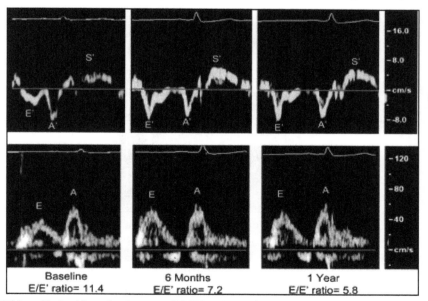

Fig. 9. Sildenafil significantly decreased E/E' at 6 months and 1 year of active treatment in patients with stable systolic heart failure

compared with placebo (P<0.01). Additionally, diastolic measures of LV function demonstrated systematic and sustained improvement after both 6 months and 1 year of sildenafil treatment. The transmitral E/A ratio, isovolumic relaxation time, and both lateral and septal E/E' decreased from baseline through 12 months (all P<0.01), which is indicative of an improvement in LV diastolic function and a decrease in LV filling pressure. Furthermore, septal T E-E' was significantly reduced at 6 and 12 months of sildenafil treatment (P<0.01). All these changes were in agreement with the observed reverse remodeling on LAVI, which is viewed as morphological expression of LV end-diastolic pressure (Lester et al., 2008). Changes observed at 6 months and 1 year after sildenafil were significantly different compared with the placebo group (P<0.01).

7. Concluding remarks

With the advancement in the management of patients with cardiovascular disease and improvement in survival following cardiovascular events, the incidence of heart failure, especially in patients of age 65 and older is increasing. Using state-of-the-art echocardiography, we and others have demonstrated that treatment with PDE-5 inhibitors improve LV function in various models of myocardial dysfunction and heart failure. These studies suggest that PDE-5 inhibitors are immensely promising for further development as novel drug therapies for myocardial infarction, LV hypertrophy and dysfunction, doxorubicin-induced cardiotoxicity, and heart failure. Clinical studies of sildenafil on heart failure patients have reported improved exercise capacity, coupled with reduced pulmonary vascular resistance and better endothelial function (Lewis et al., 2007; Guazzi et al., 2007). Sildenafil also preserved LV function in patients with heart failure due to various etiologies (Guazzi et al., 2011). Several other studies indicated that PDE-5 inhibition with sildenafil has a therapeutic promise for stroke, neurodegenerative diseases and potentially other circulatory disorders (reviewed in Kukreja et al., 2007; Kukreja et al., 2011a; Kukreja et al. 2011b). These drugs may not only delay or reduce the pathological damage or defects in various vital organs, but also improve the overall well-being and quality of life in patients.

8. Acknowledgment

This work was supported by grants from the National Institutes of Health (HL51045, HL79424 and HL93685) to Rakesh C. Kukreja and a National Scientist Development Grant from the American Heart Association (10SDG3770011) to Fadi N. Salloum.

9. References

Adamo CM. Phosphodiesterases as Drug Targets, Evaluation of the Therapeutic Utility of Phosphodiesterase 5A Inhibition in the mdx Mouse Model of Duchenne Muscular Dystrophy, eds Schmidt HHW, Hofmann F, Stasch JP (Springer-Verlag, New York). *Handbook of Experimental Pharmacology*. 2010, 192.

Adamo CM, Dai DF, Percival JM, Minami E, Willis MS, Patrucco E, Froehner SC, Beavo JA. Sildenafil reverses cardiac dysfunction in the mdx mouse model of Duchenne muscular dystrophy. *Proc Natl Acad Sci U S A*. 2010; 107:19079-83.

Anversa, P, Li P, Zhang X, Olivetti G, Capasso JM. Ischaemic myocardial injury and ventricular remodelling. *Cardiovasc Res*. 1993; 27:145-57.

Bahler RC, Mohyuddin T, Finkelhor RS, Jacobs IB. Contribution of Doppler tissue imaging and myocardial performance index to assessment of left ventricular function in patients with Duchenne's muscular dystrophy. *J Am Soc Echocardiogr.* 2005; 18:666–673.

Bremer YA, Salloum F, Ockaili R, Chou E, Moskowitz WB, Kukreja RC. Sildenafil citrate (Viagra) induces cardioprotective effects after ischemia/reperfusion injury in infant rabbits. *Pediatr Res.* 2005; 57:22-7.

Bushby K, Muntoni F, Bourke JP. 107th ENMC international workshop: The management of cardiac involvement in muscular dystrophy and myotonic dystrophy. 7th-9th June 2002, Naarden, the Netherlands. *Neuromuscul Disord.* 2003; 13:166–172.

Chau VQ, Salloum FN, Hoke NN, Abbate A, Kukreja RC. Mitigation of the Progression of Heart Failure with Sildenafil Involves Inhibition of RhoA/Rho-Kinase Pathway. *Am J Physiol Heart Circ Physiol.* 2011; 300:H2272-9.

Corbin, J.D., Francis, S.H.. Pharmacology of phosphodiesterase-5 inhibitors. *Int. J. Clin. Pract.* 2002; 56: 453-459.

Das A, Durrant D, Mitchell C, Mayton E, Hoke NN, Salloum FN, Park MA, Qureshi I, Lee R, Dent P and Kukreja RC. Sildenafil Increases Chemotherapeutic Efficacy of Doxorubicin in Prostate Cancer and Ameliorates Cardiac Dysfunction. *Proc Natl Acad Sci U.S.A.* 2010; 107:18202-7.

Devereux RB, Reichek N. Echocardiographic determination of left ventricular mass in man: anatomic validation of the method. *Circulation.* 1977; 55:613–618.

Finsterer J, Stöllberger C. The heart in human dystrophinopathies. *Cardiology.* 2003; 99:1–19.

Fisher PW, Salloum F, Das A, Hyder S, Kukreja RC. Phosphodiesterase 5A inhibition using sildenafil attenuates cardiomyocyte apoptosis and left ventricular dysfunction in chronic model of doxorubicin-induced cardiotoxicity. *Circulation.* 2005; 111:1601-1610.

Frey, N. & Olson, E.N. Cardiac hypertrophy: the good, the bad, and the ugly. *Annu. Rev. Physiol.* 2003; 65:45–79.

Frey, N. , Katus, H.A. , Olson, E.N. & Hill, J.A. Hypertrophy of the heart: a new therapeutic target? *Circulation.* 2004;109:1580–1589.

Guazzi M, Samaja M, Arena R, Vicenzi M, Guazzi MD. Long-term use of sildenafil in the therapeutic management of heart failure. *J Am Coll Cardiol.* 2007; 50:2145-2147.

Guazzi M, Vicenzi M, Arena R, Guazzi MD. PDE5 inhibition with sildenafil improves left ventricular diastolic function, cardiac geometry, and clinical status in patients with stable systolic heart failure: results of a 1-year, prospective, randomized, placebo-controlled study. *Circ Heart Fail.* 2011; 4:8-17.

Jearawiriyapaisarn N, Moulton HM, Sazani P, Kole R, Willis MS. Long-term improvement in mdx cardiomyopathy after therapy with peptide-conjugated morpholino oligomers. *Cardiovasc Res.* 2010; 85:444–453.

Khairallah M, Khairallah RJ, Young ME, Allen BG, Gillis MA, Danialou G, Deschepper CF, Petrof BJ, Des Rosiers C. Sildenafil and cardiomyocyte-specific cGMP signaling prevent cardiomyopathic changes associated with dystrophin deficiency. *Proc Natl Acad Sci USA.* 2008; 105:7028–7033.

Koka S, Das A, Zhu SG, Durrant D, Xi L, Kukreja RC. Long-acting phosphodiesterase-5 inhibitor tadalafil attenuates doxorubicin-induced cardiomyopathy without interfering with chemotherapeutic effect. *J Pharmacol Exp Ther.* 2010; 334:1023-30.

Kukreja RC, Salloum F, Das A, Ockaili R, Yin C, Bremer YA, Fisher PW, Wittkamp M, Hawkins J, Chou E, Kukreja AK, Wang X, Marwaha V, and Xi L. Pharmacological Preconditioning with Sildenafil: Basic Mechanisms and Clinical Implications. *Vascul Pharmacol.* 2005; 42: 219-232.

Kukreja RC, Salloum FN, and Xi L. Nonurologic Applications of Phosphodiesterase Type 5 Inhibitors. *Current Sexual Health Reports.* 2007; 4: 64-70.

Kukreja RC, Salloum FN, Das A, Koka S, Ockaili RA, Xi L. Emerging New Uses of Phosphodiesterase-5 Inhibitors in Cardiovascular Diseases. *Exp Clin Cardiol.* 2011(a); In press.

Kukreja RC, Salloum FN, Das A. Role of cGMP-Phosphodiesterase-5 Inhibition in Cardioprotective Signaling. *J Am Coll Cardiol.* 2011(b); In press.

Laties, A.M., Fraunfelder, F.T. Ocular safety of Viagra (sildenafil citrate). *Trans Am. Ophthalmol. Soc.* 1999; 97:115-128.

Lester SJ, Tajik AJ, Nishimura RA, Oh JK, Khandheria BK, Seward JB. Unlocking the mysteries of diastolic function: deciphering the Rosetta Stone 10 years later. *J Am Coll Cardiol.* 2008; 51:679-689.

Lewis GD, Lachmann J, camuso J, Lepore JJ, Shin J, Martinovic ME, Systrom DM, Bloch KD, Semigran MJ. Sildenafil improves exercise hemodynamics and oxygen uptake in patients with systolic heart failure. *Circulation.* 2007; 115: 59-66.

Markham LW, Michelfelder EC, Border WL, Khoury PR, Spicer RL, Wong BL, Benson DW, Cripe LH. Abnormalities of diastolic function precede dilated cardiomyopathy associated with Duchenne muscular dystrophy. *J Am Soc Echocardiogr.* 2006; 19:865-871.

McNally EM. Duchenne muscular dystrophy: how bad is the heart? *Heart.* 2008; 94:976-977.

Nagayama T, Hsu S, Zhang M, Koitabashi N, Bedja D, Gabrielson KL, Takimoto E, Kass DA. Sildenafil stops progressive chamber, cellular, and molecular remodeling and improves calcium handling and function in hearts with pre-existing advanced hypertrophy caused by pressure overload. *J Am Coll Cardiol.* 2009; 53:207-15.

Ockaili R, Salloum F, Hawkins J, Kukreja RC. Sildenafil (Viagra) induces powerful cardioprotective effect via opening of mitochondrial K_{ATP} channels in rabbits. *Am J Physiol Heart Circ Physiol.* 2002; 283: H1263-69.

Pokreisz P, Vandenwijngaert S, Bito V, Van den Bergh A, Lenaerts I, Busch C, Marsboom G, Gheysens O, Vermeersch P, Biesmans L, Liu X, Gillijns H, Pellens M, Van Lommel A, Buys E, Schoonjans L, Vanhaecke J, Verbeken E, Sipido K, Herijgers P, Bloch KD, Janssens SP. Ventricular phosphodiesterase-5 expression is increased in patients with advanced heart failure and contributes to adverse ventricular remodeling after myocardial infarction in mice. *Circulation.* 2009; 119: 408-416.

Porst, H., Rosen, R., Padma-Nathan, H., Goldstein, I., Giuliano, F., Ulbrich, E., Bandel T. The efficacy and tolerability of vardenafil, a new, oral, selective phosphodiesterase type 5 inhibitor, in patients with erectile dysfunction: the first at-home clinical trial. *Int. J. Impot. Res.* 2001; 13: 192-199.

Quiñones MA, Otto CM, Stoddard M, Waggoner A, Zoghbi WA; Doppler Quantification Task Force of the Nomenclature and Standards Committee of the American Society of Echocardiography. Recommendations for quantification of Doppler echocardiography: a report from the Doppler Quantification Task Force of the

Nomenclature and Standards Committee of the American Society of Echocardiography. *J Am Soc Echocardiogr.* 2002; 15:167–184.

Salloum FN, Abbate A, Das A, Houser JE, Mudrick CA, Qureshi IZ, Hoke NN, Roy SK, Brown WR, Prabhakar S, Kukreja RC. Sildenafil (Viagra) attenuates ischemic cardiomyopathy and improves left ventricular function in mice. *Am J Physiol Heart Circ Physiol.* 2008 (a); 294: H1398-406.

Salloum FN, Abbate A, Brown WR, Ockaili RA, Hoke NN, and Kukreja RC. Phosphodiesterase-5 Inhibitors Reduce Myocardial Infarction, Apoptosis and Improve Post-Ischemic Ventricular Function in Female Mice. *J Am Coll Cardiol.* 2008 (b); 51: 178A-178A Suppl.

Salloum FN, Chau VQ, Hoke NN, Abbate A, Varma A, Ockaili RA, Toldo S, Kukreja RC. Phosphodiesterase-5 inhibitor, Tadalafil, protects against myocardial ischemia/reperfusion through protein-kinase G dependent generation of hydrogen sulfide. *Circulation.* 2009; 120:S31-6.

Salloum FN, Ockaili R, Wittkamp M, Marwaha V.R., and Kukreja R.C. Vardenafil: a Novel Type 5 Phosphodiesterase Inhibitor Reduces Myocardial Infarct Size Following Ischemia/Reperfusion Injury via Opening of Mitochondrial KATP Channels in Rabbits. *J Mol Cell Cardiol.* 2006; 40:405-11.

Salloum FN, Takenoshita Y, Ockaili RA, Daoud VP, Chou E, Yoshida K, Kukreja RC. Sildenafil and vardenafil but not nitroglycerin limit myocardial infarction through opening of mitochondrial K(ATP) channels when administered at reperfusion following ischemia in rabbits. *J Mol Cell Cardiol.* 2007; 42:453-8.

Salloum, F, Yin C, Xi L, Kukreja RC. Sildenafil induces delayed preconditioning through inducible nitric oxide synthase-dependent pathway in mouse heart. *Circ Res.* 2003; 92:595–607.

Schiller NB, Shah PM, Crawford M, DeMaria A, Devereux R, Feigenbaum H, Gutgesell H, Reichek N, Sahn D, Schnittger I. Recommendations for quantitation of the left ventricle by two-dimensional echocardiography. American Society of Echocardiography Committee on Standards, Subcommittee on Quantitation of Two-Dimensional Echocardiograms. *J Am Soc Echocardiogr.* 1989; 2:358-367.

Takimoto E, Champion HC, Li M, Belardi D, Ren S, Rodriguez ER, Bedja D, Gabrielson KL, Wang Y, Kass DA. Chronic inhibition of cyclic GMP phosphodiesterase 5A prevents and reverses cardiac hypertrophy. *Nat Med.* 2005; 11:214-22.

Townsend D, Blankinship MJ, Allen JM, Gregorevic P, Chamberlain JS, Metzger JM. Systemic administration of micro-dystrophin restores cardiac geometry and prevents dobutamine-induced cardiac pump failure. *Mol Ther.* 2007; 15:1086–1092.

Wehling M, Spencer MJ, Tidball JG. A nitric oxide synthase transgene ameliorates muscular dystrophy in mdx mice. *J Cell Biol.* 2001; 155:123–131.

Wehling-Henricks M, Jordan MC, Roos KP, Deng B, Tidball JG. Cardiomyopathy in dystrophin-deficient hearts is prevented by expression of a neuronal nitric oxide synthase transgene in the myocardium. *Hum Mol Genet.* 2005; 14:1921–1933.

7

Pulmonary Venous Flow Pattern and Atrial Fibrillation: Fact and Controversy

Toru Maruyama[1], Yousuke Kokawa[2], Hisataka Nakamura[2],
Mitsuhiro Fukata[2], Shioto Yasuda[2], Keita Odashiro[2] and Koichi Akashi[2]

[1]*Institute of Health Science and*
[2]*Department of Medicine, Kyushu University, Fukuoka*
Japan

1. Introduction

The role of echocardiography in patients with atrial fibrillation (AF) has been changing gradually according with recent advance in echocardiographic instruments and better understanding for AF. Historically, M-mode echocardiography applied to AF patients has focused on the diagnosis of underlying organic heart diseases and on the detection of left atrial (LA) thrombi. These are not surprising because AF had been the highest risk of ischemic stroke in the era of incomplete anticoagulation therapy. Thereafter, LA size, volume and functions have been foci assessed by echocardiography. These echocardiographic procedures have been conducted for prediction and prevention of recurrence of AF paroxysms (Barbier et al, 1994; Verdecchia et al, 2003; Vasan et al, 2003). Spontaneous echo contrast has also been an established B-mode echocardiographic finding with highly predictive value of ischemic stroke. After the development of Doppler echocardiography, pulmonary venous flow (PVF) evaluation is a routine laboratory investigation for patients with and without AF. The usefulness of PVF evaluation is not limited to assess LA or left ventricular (LV) functions, but has expanded to investigation of various aspects of AF (Tabata et al., 2003). PVF recording increases its usefulness when it is combined with recordings of Doppler LV inflow pattern. This article reviews the established usefulness of PVF estimation in patients with permanent AF, and then focuses on the potential usefulness of PVF assessment in AF progression, i.e., during sinus rhythm (i.e., interval of paroxysms of AF), during ongoing paroxysmal AF, and further during the long-term AF management.

2. Clinical Perspectives of AF

AF is one of the most common sustained arrhythmias in daily clinical practice. There has been a great advance in the exploration of the etiologies of AF. These are the subject of several overlapping schemes of individual pathogenesis, i.e., atrial overload and stretch, myocardial ischemia and inflammation, degeneration and subsequent fibrosis of atrial myocardium, neurohumoral or metabolic factors, and other unknown factors. Therefore, clinical presentations of AF are very broad. This arrhythmia occurs in a variety of clinical settings such as valvular heart diseases, postoperative conditions, heart failure, hypertension, metabolic syndrome, thyrotoxicosis, and so on (**Fig. 1**). Since valvular heart diseases were historically a main etiology of AF, echocardiographic attention to AF patients was mainly rheumatic valvular lesions and detection of LA thrombi or spontaneous echo contrast which is based on the local hemostatic changes due to rheologic abnormalities (Kwaan et al, 2004; Topaloglu et al, 2007). In relation to thrombus formation, LA appendage function was highlighted in that impaired appendage function leads to thrombus formation and high risk of embolic event (Donal et al, 2005). According to an increased prevalence of coronary artery diseases, AF has been encountered in acute myocardial infarction, after coronary artery bypass grafting surgery and chronic phase of ischemic heart disease and subsequent heart failure. On the other hand, AF is often observed in patients with another kind of arrhythmias (e.g., preexcitation syndrome) or noncardiac disorders (e.g., thyrotoxicosis, chronic obstructive pulmonary disease). AF is often encountered in subjects without systemic or organic heart diseases (so-called 'lone' AF). According with relative decline of rheumatic valvular diseases, terminology of 'nonvalvular' or 'nonrheumatic' AF becomes familiar. Wide spectrum in clinical features of AF sometimes makes the therapeutic decision-making difficult (Wyse & Gersh, 2004).

AF is classified by the duration in which this arrhythmia sustains (e.g., paroxysmal, persistent and permanent). Paroxysmal AF is characterized as rare or repetitive paroxysms of short-lasting AF, which often undergoes spontaneous conversion to sinus rhythm, but rhythm-control treatment is required depending on symptom and hemodynamic deterioration. Persistent AF has the possibility of termination either by antiarrhythmic drugs or by electrical defibrillation. Permanent AF does not restore to sinus rhythm spontaneously, and hence conservative therapeutic option is the rate-control strategy. AF is not only responsible for substantial morbidity and mortality, but also impairs quality of life by limited capacities of physical activity and heart rate regulation. To date, the most effective treatment for drug-refractory AF is radiofrequency catheter ablation. Pulmonary vein (PV) isolation by circumferential ablation of PV-LA junction is a promising technique to terminate AF. Despite the introduction of novel and sophisticated ablation techniques such as irrigation catheters, pericardial approach and ganglionated plexi ablation, periprocedural complications are not negligible.

AF is characterized to date as an age-dependent, progressive disease, i.e., AF prevalence increases steeply from 0.5% at age 50 to 59 years to 9.0% at age 80 to 89 years (Kannel et al., 1998). Progressive nature of this arrhythmia is evident in that AF becomes refractory to pharmacologic treatment and electrical defibrillation in proportion with the duration of sustaining AF. This is the main feature that distinguishes AF from many other kinds of clinical arrhythmia (Wijffels et al., 1995). In a few decades, the mechanisms of such progression of AF have been clarified by many basic experiments using AF animal models and clinical studies of AF patients. Remodeling of LA plays an important role in the genesis, maintenance and perpetuation of AF. LA remodeling is a concept including electrical, contractile and structural aspects. Electrical remodeling induces abbreviated and dispersed electrical refractoriness and inhomogeneous slow conduction of electrical impulse. These are considered to be an arrhythmogenic substrate, prerequisite of AF development. Electrocardiograms (ECG) in patients with AF demonstrate characteristic fibrillation (f) waves that are evident in right precordial leads. According to the progression of AF, characteristic f-waves become gradually small in amplitude and high in frequency. On the other hand, contractile remodeling provides poor LA contraction and structural remodeling causes LA dilatation. Histologically, LA myocardium in patients with AF shows infiltration of inflammatory cells, interstitial fibrosis and loss of contractile myocytes, leading to slow, fragmented and fibrillatory conduction and poor dyssynchronous LA contractions.

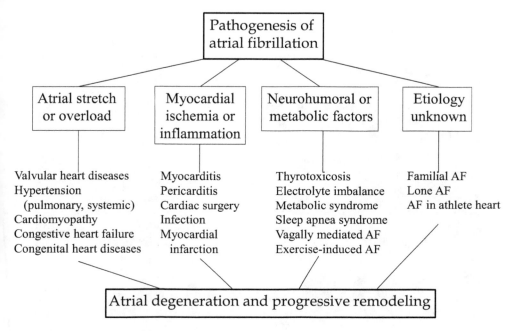

Fig. 1. Mechanisms favoring atrial fibrillation (AF).

3. Physiology of PVF

PVF recording is feasible not only by transesophageal echocardiography (TEE) but also by transthoracic echocardiography (TTE). According with the prevalence of PVF estimation by TTE, there have been investigations comparing the PVF recorded by TTE with that recorded by TEE. To date, TTE estimation of PVF is reported to provide reliable quantitation of PVF recorded by TEE in patients with and without organic heart diseases (Masuyama et al., 1995). **Fig. 2** is an actual Doppler PVF pattern during an entire cardiac cycle recorded by TTE. When ultrasound probe is positioned at the apex of chest wall, a four-chamber apical view is obtained. Then color jet is visualized in the upper LA of real-time, B-mode image. This color image is forward blood flow signals in right superior PV (**Fig. 2**, upper). After overall color Doppler interrogation, Doppler velocimetry is obtained by positioning the sampling gate 2-3 cm distal from the orifice of right superior PV (**Fig. 2**, lower).

The PVF profile is characterized as forward flows during LV systolic (**S**) and early diastolic (**D**) phases, and as reversed flow during late diastole when LA contracts (**Ar**). There are strictly two components within the **S** wave of PVF, i.e., S_1 is caused by active LA relaxation and S_2 is ascribed to passive LA wall stretching caused by vigorous LV contraction toward apical direction. Peak velocity and velocity-time integral of the **S** wave are usually greater than those of the **D** wave. Gentile et al (1997) investigated Doppler PVF parameters in 143 healthy individuals aged from 20 to 80 years by TTE. Age-dependent Doppler parameters are reported to be as follows; peak amplitude and time integral of both **S** and **D** waves, and **S/D** peak amplitude and integral ratios, whereas **Ar** wave is reported to be age-independent. These findings indicate the possibility of **Ar** wave as a diagnostic tool of various hemodynamic abnormalities in a wide range of patients' age.

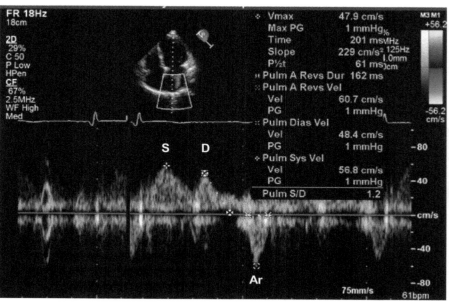

Fig. 2. Representative Doppler imaging of transthoracic echocardiography applied to a patient with hypertension. Upper image is an apical four chamber view with color flow indicating blood flow returning from right superior pulmonary vein (PV) into left atrium (LA). Middle is an ECG tracing (standard limb lead II). Lower is a continuous-wave Doppler PV flow velocimetry during an entire cardiac cycle. Upward direction indicates forward flow, whereas downward direction means reverse flow.

LA plays three different roles periodically in an entire cardiac cycle, i.e., LA acts as a 'booster pump' when LA contracts in late LV diastole, then as a 'reservoir' during LV systole, and finally as a 'conduit' during early LV diastole (**Fig. 3**). These three kinds of LA functions correspond with **Ar**, **S** and **D** waves respectively, and are estimated also by LA volume curve during an entire cardiac cycle using automatic boundary detection (Zhang et al, 1998), manual tracking (Ogawa et al, 2009), and speckle tracking techniques (Mori et al, 2011). The PVF pattern, especially **S** and **D** wave components, is influenced originally by many physiologic factors such as age, heart rate, respiration, LV function and loading conditions (Bollmann, 2007). These factors should be taken into account when evaluating PVF recording.

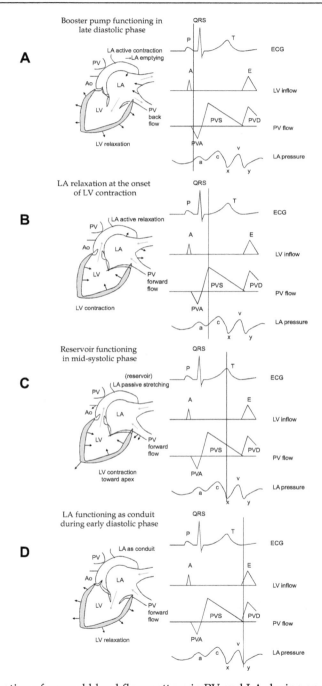

Fig. 3. Illustration of normal blood flow pattern in PV and LA during an entire cardiac cycle.

4. Myocardial sleeves in PV

In the PVF profile, **Ar** wave reflects physiologic PV regurgitation during LA contraction due to the absence of an anatomic valve at the PV-LA junction. Interestingly, PV wall contains myocardial sleeves instead of anatomic valve. **Fig. 4** is a schematic illustration of human atria and adjacent great veins. Posterior LA wall contains complicated myocardial layers for myocardial sleeves running longitudinally, cross-sectionally and obliquely within the PV walls. Histologically, myocardial sleeves exist in the mid-layer of PV walls (**Fig. 5A**). The myocardial sleeves are, therefore, considered to function as 'sphincter', which minimizes the PV regurgitation caused by LA contraction. PV contraction is actually confirmed, and this phenomenon is mainly due to the presence of myocardial sleeves contracting synchronously with LA myocardium. This is validated by radiofrequency catheter ablation, i.e., perfect PV isolation (e.g., electrical disconnection of PV-LA junction) is reported to abolish the PV contraction (Atwater et al, 2011). These sleeves also function as 'throttle' valve that regulates cardiac output for systemic circulation (Burch & Romney, 1954). The myocardial sleeves show characteristic electrophysiological properties prone to yield spontaneous repetitive firings which propagate to LA and cause frequent ectopic beats. **Fig. 5B** is the microelectrode recording of the intracellular potentials of guinea-pig LA and myocardial sleeve in PV. Resting membrane potential in myocardial sleeve is less negative relative to that of LA. Moreover, myocardial sleeve in PV show the tendency of spontaneous electrical activity leading to the abnormal automaticity initiating AF. These arrhythmogenic foci act as a 'driver' to trigger and maintain paroxysms of AF. Highly compliant PV wall allows own cyclic stretching due to physiological PV regurgitation. This phenomenon is considered to accentuate intracellular Ca^{2+} dynamics mediated by stretch-activated ion channels, which is a prerequisite of repetitive electrical firing (de Bakker et al., 2002; Honjo et al., 2003; Chou et al., 2005, Takahara et al, 2011). Moreover, the myocardial sleeves within PV show a complicated anisotropic orientation of myocardial fibers separated by fibrotic tissues causing impaired electrotonic interactions, which accentuates intrinsic spontaneous firing and triggered activity (Nathan & Eliakim, 1966).

Since Haïssaguerre et al (1998) demonstrated the ectopic and spontaneous electrical activities in the myocardial sleeves located in PV responsible for triggering AF, main stream of the AF research has been changed over the past decade, in that recent AF study focused on many areas which had not been given much attention. Importance of the myocardial sleeves as arrhythmogenic foci in AF is confirmed also in the human postmortem studies. Tagawa et al (2001) investigated myocardial sleeve distribution in patients with AF or without AF. They showed that the significantly longer distance of sleeves extending to the peripheral end of PV in AF patients relative to the distance in control patients was confirmed in inferior but not superior PV. In addition, myocytes in PV of AF patients were not uniform and surrounded by fibrous tissues compared with those in controls. Moreover, Steiner et al (2006) reported that amyloid deposition and scarring in myocardial sleeves tended to be observed more frequently in AF patients relative to control patients. Interestingly, the incidence of atrial myocardium extending beyond the PV-LA junction up to the PV periphery in all the examined PV specimens is commonly reported to be 88 to 89% (Tagawa et al, 2001; Steiner et al, 2006).

According with an advance of immunohistochemical techniques, autonomic nervous innervation in PV has been elucidated. Ganglionated plexi are reported to be abundant around the great vessels of the human heart including PV (Armour et al, 1997).

Furthermore, both cholinergic and adrenergic nerve endings are found together within a single neural plexus of PV, and nerve density is highest in the PV antrum (Tan et al, 2006). The physiological meaning of these ganglionated plexi remains to be speculative. Considering the 'throttle' valve function of myocardial sleeves, ganglionated plexi located in PV-LA junctions may play a role of neural control of cardiac output by regulating proximal PV tonus. Elevated PV tonus associated with pathological condition such as heart failure (e.g., ganglionated plexi out of neural control) may lead to the occasion of acute pulmonary edema leading to severe dyspnea or orthopnea. AF *per se* also shows potential autonomic influence (**Fig. 1**). The correlations between the neural aspect of AF and the ganglionated plexi possibly influencing PV tonus or contraction are the subjects of future study.

5. PVF during ongoing AF

PVF is visualized by Doppler echocardiography not only in sinus rhythm but also during AF. AF is characterized by electrophysiological and mechanical properties such as rapid, irregular and fragmented electrical activities and absence of complete LA contraction and relaxation. Therefore, PVF during AF is known as loss of **Ar** wave, blunted **S** wave and relatively dominant **D** wave. Loss of synchronous LA contraction is reflected by disappearance of **Ar** wave. Similarly, loss of complete LA relaxation causes a delayed onset of **S** wave.

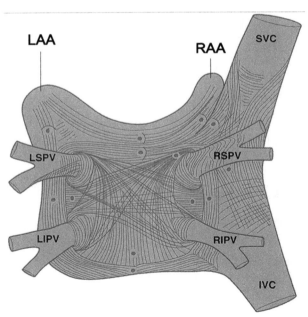

Fig. 4. Schematic illustration of human atria and adjacent great veins. Myocardial sleeves run in PV wall longitudinally, obliquely and cross-sectionally. Myocardial sleeve in superior PV is usually longer than that in inferior PV. IVC, inferior vena cava; LAA, left atrial appendage; LIPV, left inferior PV; LSPV, left superior PV; RAA, right atrial appendage; RIPV, right inferior PV; RSPV, right superior PV; SVC, superior vena cava.

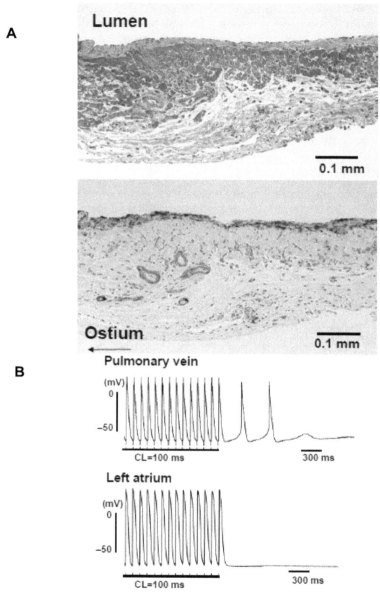

Fig. 5. **A:** Microscopic findings of PV obtained from guinea pig (upper: masson trichrome staining, lower: immunostaining for α-smooth muscle actin). **B:** Electrophysiological characteristics of PV and LA. (From Takahara, A.; Sugimoto, T.; Kitamura, T.; Takeda, K.; Tsuneoka, Y.; Namekata, I. & Tanaka, H. Electrophysiological and pharmacological characteristics of triggered activity elicited in guinea-pig pulmonary vein myocardium. *Journal of Pharmacological Science* Vol. 115, No. 2, 2011, pp. 176-181, with permission.)

This phenomenon is due to loss of S_1 wave that reflects forward PV flow under the active LA relaxation. Moreover, early systolic reversed PVF is sometimes observed (Tabata et al., 2003; Bollmann, 2007). This is reflected by reversed PV-LA pressure gradient at this moment of the early systolic phase. S_2 *per se* is also blunted under the increased LA stiffness during AF. LA functions of 'reservoir' and 'booster pump' are impaired profoundly under the presence of AF. Impaired LA functions result in the reduction of stroke volume by 38% even in AF patients without organic heart diseases (Alboni et al, 1995). Therefore, only the 'conduit' function of LA remains, which leads to the greater **D** wave relative to S_2 wave (Chao et al., 2000). These echocardiographic findings are important predictors of progressive LA remodeling.

6. PVF during sinus rhythm in AF patients

AF is a progressive disease showing electrical, contractile and structural LA remodeling (Wijffels et al., 1995). It is well known that paroxysms of AF gradually become refractory to pharmacologic treatment and electrical defibrillation. Accordingly, paroxysmal AF becomes persistent AF, and finally converts to permanent AF, although individual difference in such time course exists. For sonographers and cardiologists, one of the greatest echocardiographic interests during sinus rhythm in AF patients is to predict future paroxysms and progression of AF. Conventionally, prediction of AF progression is based mainly on LA size, volume, and functions (Barbier et al, 1994; Verdecchia et al, 2003; Vasan et al, 2003). Such evaluations have been performed historically by various echocardiographic techniques such as M-mode measurement, LV inflow Doppler velocimetry, strain-rate imaging, three-dimensional echocardiography speckle tracking technique and so on. Two-dimensional speckle tracking echocardiography monitors LA volume curve during an entire cardiac cycle, which enables accurate evaluations of aforementioned three kinds of LA functions (e.g., 'reservoir', 'conduit' and 'booster pump' functions). This technique showed reduced 'reservoir' and 'booster pump' functions in patients with paroxysmal AF (Mori et al., 2011).

PVF recording in sinus rhythm of AF patients has been receiving increasing attention, because 'focal' AF originates predominantly from PV (Haïssaguerre et al., 1998), and wide spectrum of paroxysmal to persistent AF associated with and without organic heart diseases shows similar characteristics of 'focal' AF. PV orifice morphologies in conjunction with AF progression have been investigated over the years by various modalities such as TEE (Knackstedt et al, 2003), magnetic resonance (MR) imaging (Tsao et al, 2001; Takase et al., 2004) and multislice computed tomography (Scharf et al, 2003). These investigations have been conducted under the uniform hypothesis that largest PV is the main source of ectopic electrical activities triggering and sustaining AF. **Fig. 6** demonstrates the PV images obtained by MR angiography applied to the patients with paroxysmal (**Fig. 6A**) or permanent (**Fig. 6B**) AF and with sinus rhythm (**Fig. 6C**). Four PV diameters are reported to be greater in the order of patients with permanent AF > those with paroxysmal AF > those with sinus rhythm (Takase et al., 2004). Moreover, PV branching pattern observed in AF patients is complicated compared with that of patients with sinus rhythm. These indicate that most permanent and paroxysmal AF stems from 'focal' AF, and that progressive structural remodeling caused by AF affects both LA and PV. With respect to the PV/LA diameter ratio, there has been a controversy, i.e., this ratio in patients with AF tended to be greater than that of patients without AF (Knackstedt et al, 2003), whereas this ratio was the same among the patient groups of paroxysmal AF, permanent AF and sinus rhythm (Tsao et al, 2001). These discrepant results may be attributed in part to the different imaging modalities and AF patients' enrollment.

In spite of accumulated morphological investigations of PV-LA junction in AF patients, there have been controversies in echocardiographic PVF patterns during sinus rhythm in patients susceptible to AF. Kosmala et al (2006) reported that an abnormal PVF pattern was observed in patients with AF, i.e., abbreviated acceleration time and prolonged deceleration time in **S** wave, indicating impaired LA relaxation and compliance. Similarly, Lindgren et al (2003) reported the reduced **S** wave amplitude as a predictor of AF progression. These are compatible to the findings reported by two-dimensional speckle tracking method (Mori et al, 2011). On the other hand, increased **Ar** wave amplitude in sinus rhythm is reported to be a potential marker of AF progression in hypertensive patients in our laboratory (**Fig. 7**). **Ar** amplitude and velocity-time integral of **Ar** wave are supposed to be linked closely to the sphincter function of myocardial sleeves located in PV (**Fig. 4**, **Fig. 5A**), i.e., impaired sphincter function theoretically allows more PV regurgitation and **Ar** wave augmentation. Surprisingly, increased **Ar** amplitude is associated with reduced, but not increased, LA contractility in our study (Maruyama et al, 2008). These findings imply that PV sphincter dysfunction is linked to the contractile LA remodeling responsible for AF progression. LA contractile performance is usually quantified as LA fractional shortening (LAFS), which is calculated by the following equation (**Fig. 8**),

$$LAFS = (LADa - LADd) / LADa \qquad (1)$$

where, LADa is an LA diameter at the beginning of LA contraction, and LADd is a minimum LA diameter during active LA contraction (Barbier et al, 1994). This is a simple measure of LA contractility obtained by M-mode echocardiography, although it is a parameter estimated only in the anteroposterior LA direction. **Ar** wave augmentation is associated with reduced LAFS, and predictive values of PV regurgitation (e.g., peak PV backflow velocity: PVBV), LA contractile function (e.g., LAFS) and LA size (e.g., LADd) for AF progression are assessed. Consequently, receiver-operating curve (ROC) indicated that the amplitude of age-independent **Ar** wave (e.g., PVBV) showed the greatest predictive value for the perpetuation of AF (**Fig. 9**). So far, the reason for discrepant results showing the importance of impaired forward flow (**S** wave) vs. augmented backward flow (**Ar** wave) in AF progression is unknown. PV regurgitation reflected by augmented **Ar** wave amplitude (e.g., PVBV) is determined by LA-PV pressure gradient (e.g., balance between LA contractile function and PV 'sphincter' function). These structures are under the influence of continuous remodeling according to the AF progression, which differs in individual AF patient. There are so many echocardiographic indices with different sensitivities and specificities. Echocardiography recorded during sinus rhythm at different stages of long-term AF progression may have resulted in such discrepant outcomes. Therefore, in personal opinion, it seems uncertain whether or not such comparisons of echocardiographic investigations are meaningful or fruitful.

Ar wave augmentation indicating an extent of PV regurgitation is considered to be a PV remodeling based on the impaired 'sphincter' function of the myocardial sleeves surrounding the PV-LA junction (**Fig. 4, Fig. 5A**). This is considered to be due to the histological, electrical and mechanical abnormalities of the myocardial sleeves. On the other hand, reduced LAFS means the contractile LA remodeling, and increased LADd reflects

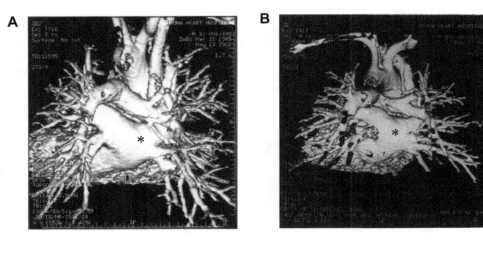

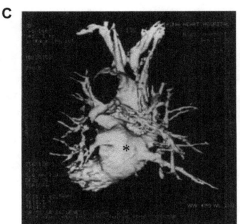

Fig. 6. Representative magnetic resonance angiography of patients with paroxysmal (**A**) or permanent (**B**) AF and with sinus rhythm (**C**). Diameters of pulmonary veins in AF patients are greater than those in patients with sinus rhythm. Landmark (*) showing the center of posterior wall of left atrium was indicated. (From Takase, B.; Nagata, M.; Matsui, T.; Kihara, T.; Kameyama, A.; Hamabe, A.; Noya, K.; Satomura, K.; Ishihara, M.; Kurita, A. & Ohsuzu, F. Pulmonary vein dimensions and variation of branching pattern in patients with paroxysmal atrial fibrillation using magnetic resonance angiography. *Japanese Heart Journal* Vol. 45, No. 1, 2004, pp. 81-92, with permission.)

in part the structural LA remodeling. It is, therefore, of interest which part of remodeling shows the greatest influence on the AF progression and perpetuation. In our study, PV remodeling demonstrated the greatest influence on the perpetuation of AF by the ROC analysis (**Fig. 9**). Knackstedt et al (2003) reported no correlation between PV diameter and LA size in patients with or without AF. Considering their TEE study, PV remodeling (e.g., dilation and regurgitation) plays a key role in AF progression (Scharf et al, 2003), although it is uncertain whether PV remodeling is a cause or a consequence of AF progression. PV wall is relatively more compliant and hence more susceptible to hemodynamics altered by paroxysms of AF than LA wall. Therefore, in personal opinion, these vessel properties of PV relates to susceptibility to AF-induced remodeling.

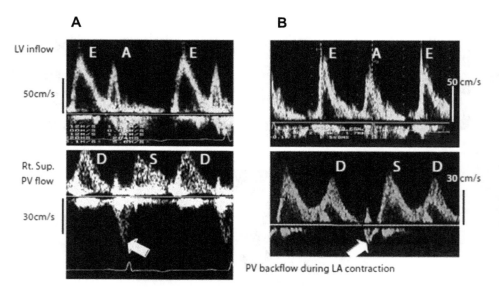

Fig. 7. Representative pulsed-wave Doppler findings of time-matched LV inflow (upper) and right superior pulmonary vein (PV) flow patterns (lower) during sinus rhythm in patients with AF which became permanent (**A**) or remained paroxysmal (**B**). Peak velocity of PV backflow (**Ar** wave) during left atrial (LA) contraction in **A** (left white arrow) was obviously greater than that in **B** (right white arrow). Time-integral of PV backflow in **A** is also greater than that in **B**. Note that scale in LV inflow is different from that in PV flow. (From Maruyama, T.; Kishikawa, T.; Ito, H.; Kaji, Y.; Sasaki, Y. & Ishihara, Y. Augmentation of pulmonary vein backflow velocity during left atrial contraction: a novel phenomenon responsible for progression of atrial fibrillation in hypertensive patients. *Cardiology* Vol. 109, No. 1, 2008, pp. 33-40, with permission.)

After the termination of AF episode, LA contractile function is briefly impaired. This impairment is gradually restored, and this reversible phenomenon is well known as LA stunning. One of the main causes of this stunning is considered to be based on the intracellular handling of cytosolic Ca^{2+}, which is important in cardiac performance but disturbed during AF. The aspects of atrial cardiomyopathy induced by tachycardia and atrial hibernation or fibrosis are also involved in the genesis of LA stunning (Khan, 2003). Recovery from LA stunning depends on the duration of AF, mode of defibrillation, and LA size, i.e., AF lasting 10 to 20 minutes does not cause observable stunning (Sparks et al, 1999) and recovery of LA contractile function is early in the order of spontaneous conversion to sinus rhythm > pharmacological defibrillation > electrical defibrillation. AF patients with normal LA size are also apt to show earlier LA functional recovery (Mattioli et al, 1998; Khan, 2003).

Thromboembolic event is a major complication of AF. This complication after defibrillation has been attributed to the dislodgement of LA thrombi during the recovery from LA stunning. Therefore, serial echocardiographic investigation and optimal anticoagulation treatment are necessary during this period. LA stunning is observed also in the case of AF treated with radiofrequency catheter ablation. Stavrakis et al (2011) investigated the acute changes of LA function and PVF pattern following PV isolation associated with ganglionated plexi ablation by TEE. They reported augmentation of both **D** and **S** waves, decrease of **S/D** ratio, and trend toward an increase in LA appendage emptying velocities after the ablation. LA appendage emptying velocity closely relates to LA stunning, and reduced **S/D** ratio reflects impaired LA relaxation in the postablative period. These TEE findings are consistent with those reported by Lindgren et al (2003) in the paroxysmal interval of AF patients.

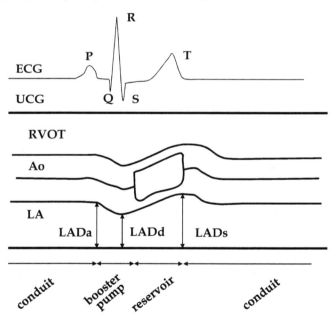

Fig. 8. Schematic illustration of the M-mode estimation of left atrial (LA) contractile function. LA dimension is variable depending on cardiac cycle. LADa, LA dimension immediately prior to the onset of LA contraction; LADd, minimal LA dimension at the end of the active LA contraction; LADs, maximal LA dimension at the end-systole. LA fractional shortening (LAFS) is calculated by equation (1) in the text. LA plays three kinds of hemodynamic function during an entire cardiac cycle (text). Aortic valve opening time corresponds to the left ventricular ejection period. Ao, aortic root; ECG, electrocardiogram; RVOT, right ventricular outflow tract; UCG, ultrasound cardiogram.

7. PVF in AF management

Pharmacological AF management is mainly divided into rhythm control and rate control strategies, both of which show equivalent outcomes in long-term prognosis of AF patients provided that appropriate anticoagulation therapy is conducted (Wyse, 2005). However, choice of better strategy based only on electrophysiologic or electrocardiographic perspectives seems insufficient. PVF evaluation has the potential to play a role in this decision-making process, i.e., PVF recording enables evaluation of contractile LA and PV functions, which vary during the long period of AF remodeling affecting both LA and PV. For AF management, it is important to assess the stage of AF progression in individual AF patient with different clinical background. For this purpose, assessment of LA stiffness or contractility and severity of PV regurgitation by PVF profile is important for AF management in individual patient.

Radiofrequency catheter ablation is widely conducted in many electrophysiologic laboratories. It is a first line therapy for 'focal' AF originating from PV, and is currently applied not only to paroxysmal AF but also to persistent AF. Remodeling makes AF drug-refractory. Moreover, antiarrhythmic drugs often suppress cardiac performance (negative inotropism) and are sometimes arrhythmogenic (proarrhythmic effects). The main

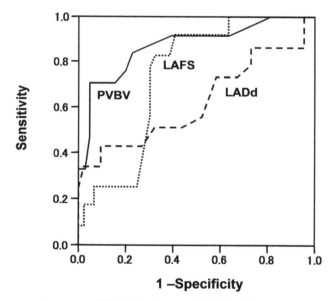

Fig. 9. Receiver-operating curve (ROC) discriminated PV backflow velocity (PVBV) as the best predictor of the progression of AF. Areas under the ROC for PVBV, left atrial fractional shortening (LAFS) and left atrial diameter at end-diastole (LADd) are 0.873, 0.740 and 0.623, respectively. Cut-off PVBV for predicting future AF perpetuation is 21.8 cm/sec (sensitivity 84.6%, specificity 78.3%). LAFS is calculated by equation (1) in the text. (From Maruyama, T.; Kishikawa, T.; Ito, H.; Kaji, Y.; Sasaki, Y. & Ishihara, Y. Augmentation of pulmonary vein backflow velocity during left atrial contraction: a novel phenomenon responsible for progression of atrial fibrillation in hypertensive patients. *Cardiology* Vol. 109, No. 1, 2008, pp. 33-40, with permission.)

procedure for ablation is electrical isolation of PV-LA junctions, i.e., disconnection of arrhythmogenic PV and adjacent antrum. Although recent advance in navigation system and new catheter device have enabled safe and effective PV isolation, PV stenosis remains a major complication especially of circumferential PV isolation. Pulmonary veno-occlusive syndrome associated with secondary pulmonary hypertension is a serious late-onset complication. During this procedure, mild-to-moderate forward PVF (e.g., **S** and **D** waves) acceleration is recorded, but this acceleration is transient and well tolerated (Ren et al., 2002). PVF monitoring is a practical and cost-effective method for early detection of this serious complication (Tabata et al., 2003; Bollmann 2007). When considering PVF is influenced by heart rate and autonomic tone (Ren et al., 2004), computed tomography or MR imaging is required to determine the therapeutic indication for balloon dilatation of PV stenosis.

8. PVF and AF progression

All the components of PVF have the potential role to evaluate AF progression, i.e., **S** wave attenuation and consequent relative **D** wave augmentation indicate impaired LA relaxation and compliance. Considering increased **D** and **Ar** wave amplitudes during sinus rhythm in AF patients, PVF increases exclusively during LV diastole, whichever PVF direction is forward (e.g., **D** wave) or backward (e.g., **Ar** wave). If ectopic beats originating from PV are mechanically triggered, these echocardiographic findings indicate that ectopic beats are prone to occur during diastole. Therefore, repetitive PV ectopic beats easily capture ventricles that are out of refractory period, and induce rapid ventricular response during 'focal' AF. This is important because rapid AF is easy to promote electrical remodeling (Wijffels et al., 1995).

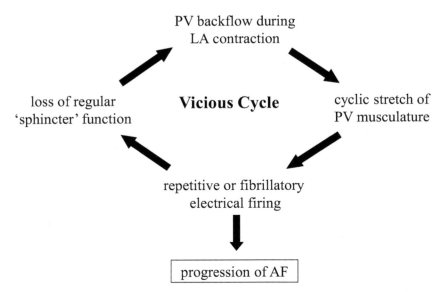

Fig. 10. Possible mechanisms of reversed PV flow (**Ar** wave) augmentation contributing to the AF progression.

AF progression is reported to be associated with greater PV diameter (Knackstedt et al., 2003; Tsao et al., 2001) as a consequence of PV remodeling (Scharf et al., 2003). Although the relation of AF and PV contraction remains to be fully investigated, augmentation of **Ar** wave (e.g., PVBV) may cause cyclic stretching of highly compliant myocardial sleeves in PV, repetitive ectopic beats and loss of 'sphincter' function, which underlie further PV regurgitation. Therefore, **D** and **Ar** waves augmentation, PV myocardial sleeve stretching and ectopic beats form a vicious cycle leading to PV remodeling. A possible mechanism by which PV characteristics contribute to AF progression is demonstrated in **Fig. 10**.

9. Conclusion

AF is the most common clinical arrhythmia showing progressive features. There has been evidence to suggest PV as a source of abnormal electrical activities initiating and sustaining AF. Currently, PVF recording is feasible in routine Doppler echocardiography, and is essential for evaluation of LA functioning three roles during an entire cardiac cycle such as 'booster pump', 'reservoir' and 'conduit'. This flow pattern recognition is of clinical importance not only in assessing global cardiac performance but also for obtaining considerable information with respect to the pathophysiology and management of AF. There has been a consensus with respect to the PVF pattern during ongoing AF or in patients with permanent AF. However, there has been a controversy concerning PVF profile during sinus rhythm in patients with paroxysmal AF. This indicates the anatomical and pathophysiological complexities of PV-LA junction and AF itself. Time-dependent recovery of LA contractile function (LA stunning) and neuroanatomical modification of PV-LA junction by radiofrequency catheter ablation make this controversy further complicated. In spite of such controversy and complexity, PVF recording has potential benefits to assess various stages of long-term AF progression and to manage the AF patients.

10. Acknowledgements

The authors thank the echocardiographic laboratory staff in Kyushu University Hospital, Fukuoka, Japan for contribution to this work.

11. References

Alboni, P.; Scarfò, S.; Fucà, G.; Paparella, N. & Yannacopulu, P. (1995). Hemodynamics of idiopathic paroxysmal atrial fibrillation. *Pacing and Clinical Electrophysiology* Vol. 18. No. 5 (Pt 1), (May 1995), pp. 980-985, ISSN 0147-8389

Armour, JA.; Murphy, DA.; Yuan, BX.; Macdonald, S. & Hopkins, DA. (1997). Gross and microscopic anatomy of the human intrinsic cardiac nervous system. *The Anatomical Record* Vol. 247, No. 2, (February 1997), pp. 289-298, ISSN 1932-8494

Atwater, BD.; Wallace, TW.; Kim, HW.; Hranitzky, PM.; Bahnson, TD.; Hegland, DD. & Daubert, JP. (2011). Pulmonary vein contraction before and after radiofrequency ablation for atrial fibrillation. *Journal of Cardiovasuclar Electrophysiology* Vol. 22, No. 2, (February 2011), pp. 169-174, ISSN 1540-8167

Barbier, P.; Alioto, G. & Guazzi, MD. (1994). Left atrial function and ventricular filling in hypertensive patients with paroxysmal atrial fibrillation. *Journal of the American College of Cardiology* Vol. 24, No. 1, (July 1994), pp. 165-170, ISSN 0735-1097

Bollmann, A. (2007). Pulmonary venous flow assessed by Doppler echocardiography in the management of atrial fibrillation (Review). *Echocardiography* Vol. 24, No. 4, (April 2007), pp. 430-435, ISSN 1540-8175

Burch, GE. & Romney, RB. (1954). Functional anatomy and throttle valve action on the pulmonary veins. *American Heart Journal* Vol. 47, No. 1, (January 1954), pp. 58-66, ISSN 0002-8703

Chao, TH.; Tsai, LM.; Tsai, WC.; Li, YH.; Lin, LJ. & Chen, JH. (2000). Effects of atrial fibrillation on pulmonary venous flow patterns assessed by Doppler transesophageal echocardiography. *Chest* Vol. 117, No. 6, (June 2000), pp. 1546-1550, ISSN 0012-3692

Chou, CC.; Nihei, M.; Zhou, S.; Tan, S.; Kawase, A.; Macias, ES.; Fishbein, MC.; Lin, SF. & Chen, PS. (2005). Intracellular calcium dynamics and anisotropic reentry in isolated canine pulmonary veins and left atrium. *Circulation* Vol. 111, No. 22, (June 2005), pp. 2889-2897, ISSN 0009-7322

de Bakker, JMT.; Ho, SY. & Hocini, M. (2002). Basic and clinical electrophysiology of pulmonary vein ectopy (Review). *Cardiovascular Research* Vol. 54, No. 2, (May 2002), pp. 287-294, ISSN 0008-6363

Donal, E.; Yamada, H.; Leclercq, C. & Herpin, D. (2005). The left atrial appendage, a small, blind-ended structure: a review of its echocardiographic evaluation and its clinical role (Review). *Chest* Vol. 128, No. 3, (September 2005), pp. 1853-1862, ISSN 0012-3692

Gentile, F.; Mantero, A.; Lippolis, A.; Ornaghi, M.; Azzollini, M.; Barbier, P.; Beretta, L.; Casazza, F.; Corno, R.; Faletra, F.; Giagnoni, E.; Gualtierotti, C.; Lombroso, S.; Mattioli, R.; Morabito, A.; Pegi, M.; Todd, S. & Pezzano, A. (1997). Pulmonary venous flow velocity patterns in 143 normal subjects aged 20 to 80 years old: an echo 2D colour Doppler cooperative study. *European Heart Journal* Vol. 18, No. 1, (January 1997), pp. 148-164, ISSN 0195-668X

Haïssaguerre, M.; Jaïs, P.; Shah, DC.; Takahashi, A.; Hocini, M.; Quiniou, G.; Garrigue, S.; Le Mouroux, A.; Le Metayer, P. & Clémenty, J. (1998). Spontaneous initiation of atrial fibrillation by ectopic beats originating in the pulmonary veins. *New England Journal of Medicine* Vol. 339, No. 10, (September 1998), pp. 659-666, ISSN 0028-4793

Honjo, H.; Boyett, MR.; Niwa, R.; Inada, S.; Yamamoto, M.; Mitsui, K.; Horiuchi, T.; Shibata, N.; Kamiya, K. & Kodama, I. (2003). Pacing-induced spontaneous activity in myocardial sleeves of pulmonary veins after treatment with ryanodine. *Circulation* Vol. 107, No. 14, (April 2003), pp. 1937-1943, ISSN 0009-7322

Kannel, WB.; Wolf, PA.; Benjamin, EJ. & Levy, D. (1998). Prevalence, incidence, prognosis, and predisposing conditions for atrial fibrillation: population-based estimates. *American Journal of Cardiology* Vol. 82, Supplement 8A, (October 1998), pp. 2N-9N, ISSN 0002-9149

Khan, IA. (2003). Atrial stunning: determinants and cellular mechanisms. *American Heart Journal* Vol. 145, No. 5, (May 2003), pp. 787-794, ISSN 0002-8703

Knackstedt, C.; Visser, L.; Plisiene, J.; Zarse, M.; Waldmann, M.; Mischke, K.; Koch, KC.; Hoffmann, R.; Franke, A.; Hanrath, P. & Schauerte, P. (2003). Dilatation of the pulmonary veins in atrial fibrillation: a transesophageal echocardiographic evaluation. *Pacing and Clinical Electrophysiology* Vol. 26, No. 6, (June 2003), pp. 1371-1378, ISSN 0147-8389

Kosmala, W.; Przewlocka-Kosmala, M. & Mazurek, W. (2006). Abnormalities of pulmonary venous flow in patients with lone atrial fibrillation. *Europace* Vol. 8, No. 2, (February 2006), pp.102-106, ISSN 1099-5129

Kwaan, HC.; Sakurai, S. & Wang, J. (2003). Rheological abnormalities and thromboembolic complications in heart disease: spontaneous echo contrast and red cell aggregation (Review). *Seminars in Thrombosis and Hemostasis* Vol. 29, No. 5, (October 2003), pp. 529-534, ISSN 0094-6176

Lindgren, KS.; Pekka Raatikainen, MJ.; Juhani Airaksinen, KE. & Huikuri, HV. (2003). Relationship between the frequency of paroxysmal episodes of atrial fibrillation and pulmonary venous flow pattern. *Europace* Vol. 5, No. 1, (January 2003), pp. 17-23, ISSN 1099-5129

Maruyama, T.; Kishikawa, T.; Ito, H.; Kaji, Y.; Sasaki, Y. & Ishihara, Y. (2008). Augmentation of pulmonary vein backflow velocity during left atrial contraction: a novel phenomenon responsible for progression of atrial fibrillation in hypertensive patients. *Cardiology* Vol. 109, No. 1, (January 2008), pp. 33-40, ISSN 0008-6312

Masuyama, T.; Nagano, R.; Nariyama, K.; Lee, JM.; Yamamoto, K.; Naito, J.; Mano, T.; Kondo, H.; Hori, M. & Kamada, T. (1995). Transthoracic Doppler echocardiographic measurements of pulmonary venous flow velocity patterns: comparison with transesophageal measurements. *Journal of the American Society of Echocardiography* Vol. 8, No. 1, (January-February 1995), pp. 61-69, ISSN 0894-7317

Mattioli, AV.; Castelli, A.; Andria, A. & Mattioli, G. (1998). Clinical and echocardiographic features influencing recovery of atrial function after cardioversion of atrial fibrillation. *Amerian Journal of Cardiology* Vol. 82, No. 11, (December 1998), pp. 1368-1371, ISSN 0002-9149

Mori, M.; Kanzaki, H.; Amaki, M.; Ohara, T.; Hasegawa, T.; Takahama, H.; Hashimura, K.; Konno, T.; Hayashi, K.; Yamagishi, M. & Kitakaze, M. (2011). Impact of reduced left atrial functions on diagnosis of paroxysmal atrial fibrillation: results from analysis of time-left atrial volume curve determined by two-dimensional speckle tracking. *Journal of Cardiology* Vol. 57, No. 1, (January 2011), pp. 89-94, ISSN 0914-5087

Nathan, H. & Eliakim, M. (1966). The junction between the left atrium and the pulmonary veins: an anatomic study of human hearts. *Circulation* Vol. 34, No. 3, (September 1966), pp. 412-422, ISSN 0009-7322

Ogawa, K.; Hozumi, T.; Sugioka, K.; Iwata, S.; Otsuka, R.; Takagi, Y.; Yoshitani, H.; Yoshiyama, M. & Yoshikawa, J. (2009). Automated assessment of left atrial function from time-left atrial volume curves using a novel speckle tracking imaging method. *Journal of the American Society of Echocardiography* Vol. 22, No. 1, (January 2009), pp. 63-69, ISSN 0894-7317

Ren, JF.; Marchlinski, FE.; Callans, DJ. & Zado, ES. (2002). Intracardiac Doppler echocardiographic quantification of pulmonary vein flow velocity: an effective technique for monitoring pulmonary vein ostia narrowing during focal atrial fibrillation ablation. *Journal of Cardiovascular Electrophysiology* Vol. 13, No. 11, (November 2002), pp. 1076-1081, ISSN 1540-8167

Ren, JF.; Marchlinski, FE. & Callans, DJ. (2004). Effect of heart rate and isoproterenol on pulmonary vein flow velocity following radiofrequency ablation: a Doppler color flow imaging study. *Journal of Interventional Cardiac Electrophysiology* Vol. 10, No. 3, (June 2004), pp. 265-269, ISSN 1383-875X

Scharf, C.; Sneider, M.; Case, I.; Chugh, A.; Lai, SW.; Pelosi, F.; Knight, BP.; Kazerooni, E.; Morady, F. & Oral, H. (2003). Anatomy of the pulmonary veins in patients with atrial fibrillation and effects of segmental ostial ablation analyzed by computed tomography. *Journal of Cardiovascular Electrophysiology* Vol. 14, No. 2, (February 2003), pp. 150-155, ISSN 1540-8167

Sparks, PB.; Jayaprakash, S.; Mond, HG.; Vohra, JK.; Grigg, LE. & Kalman, JM. (1999). Left atrial mechanical function after brief duration atrial fibrillation. *Journal of the American College of Cardiology* Vol. 33, No. 2, (February 1999), pp. 342-349, ISSN 0735-1097

Stavrakis, S.; Madden, G.; Pokharel, D.; Po, SS.; Nakagawa, H.; Jackman, WM. & Sivaram, CA. (2011). Transesophageal echocardiographic assessment of pulmonary veins and left atrium in patients undergoing atrial fibrillation ablation. *Echocardiography* Vol. 28, No. 7, (August 2011), pp. 775-781, ISSN 1540-8175

Steiner, I.; Hájková, P.; Kvasnička, J. & Kholová, I. (2006). Myocardial sleeves of pulmonary veins and atrial fibrillation: a postmortem histopathological study of 100 subjects. *Virchows Archiv* Vol. 449, No. 1, (July 2006), pp. 88-95, ISSN 0945-6317

Tabata, T.; Thomas, JD. & Klein, AL. (2003). Pulmonary venous flow by Doppler echocardiography: revisited 12 years later. *Journal of the American College of Cardiology* Vol. 41, No. 8, (April 2003), pp. 1243-1250, ISSN 0735-1097

Tagawa, M.; Higuchi, K.; Chinushi, M.; Washizuka, T.; Ushiki, T.; Ishihara, N. & Aizawa, Y. (2001). Myocardium extending from the left atrium onto the pulmonary veins: a comparison between subjects with and without atrial fibrillation. *Pacing and Clinical Electrophysiology* Vol. 24, No. 10, (October 2001), pp. 1459-1463, ISSN 0147-8389

Takahara, A.; Sugimoto, T.; Kitamura, T.; Takeda, K.; Tsuneoka, Y.; Namekata, I. & Tanaka, H. (2011). Electrophysiological and pharmacological characteristics of triggered activity elicited in guinea-pig pulmonary vein myocardium. *Journal of Pharmacological Science* Vol. 115, No. 2, (February 2011), pp. 176-181, ISSN 1347-8613

Takase, B.; Nagata, M.; Matsui, T.; Kihara, T.; Kameyama, A.; Hamabe, A.; Noya, K.; Satomura, K.; Ishihara, M.; Kurita, A. & Ohsuzu, F. (2004). Pulmonary vein dimensions and variation of branching pattern in patients with paroxysmal atrial fibrillation using magnetic resonance angiography. *Japanese Heart Journal* Vol. 45, No. 1, (January 2004), pp. 81-92, ISSN 0021-4868

Tan, AY.; Li, H.; Wachsmann-Hogiu, S.; Chen, LS.; Chen, PS. & Fishbein, MC. (2006). Autonomic innervation and segmental muscular disconnections at the human pulmonary vein-atrial junction: implications for catheter ablation of atrial-pulmonary vein junction. *Journal of the American College of Cardiology* Vol. 48, No. 1, (July 2006), pp. 132-143, ISSN 0735-1097

Topaloglu, S.; Boyaci, A.; Ayaz, S.; Yilmaz, S.; Yanik, O.; Ozdemir, O.; Soylu, M.; Demir, AD.; Aras, D.; Kisacik, HL. & Korkmaz, S. (2007). Coagulation, fibrinolytic system activation and endothelial dysfunction in patients with mitral stenosis and sinus rhythm. *Angiology* Vol. 58, No. 1, (February-March 2007), pp. 85-91, ISSN 0003-3197

Tsao, HM.; Yu, WC.; Cheng, HC.; Wu, MH.; Tai, CT.; Lin, WS.; Ding, YA.; Chang, MS. & Chen, SA. (2001). Pulmonary vein dilatation in patients with atrial fibrillation: detection by magnetic resonance imaging. *Journal of Cardiovascular Electrophysiology* Vol. 12, No. 7, (July 2001), pp. 809-813, ISSN 1540-8167

Vasan, RS.; Larson, MG.; Levy, D.; Galderisi, M.; Wolf, PA. & Benjamin, EJ. (2003). Doppler transmitral flow indexes and risk of atrial fibrillation (the Framingham Heart Study). *American Journal of Cardiology* Vol. 91, No. 9, (May 2003), pp. 1079-1083, ISSN 0002-9149

Verdecchia, P.; Reboldi, G.; Gattobigio, R.; Bentivoglio, M.; Borgioni, C.; Angeli, F.; Carluccio, E.; Sardone, MG. & Porcellati, C. (2003). Atrial fibrillation in hypertension: predictors and outcome. *Hypertension* Vol. 41, No. 2, (February 2003), pp. 218-223, ISSN 0194-911X

Wijffels, MC.; Kirchhof, CJ.; Dorland, R. & Allessie, MA. (1995). Atrial fibrillation begets atrial fibrillation: a study in awake chronically instrumented goats. *Circulation* Vol. 92, No. 7, (October 1995), pp. 1954-1968, ISSN 0009-7322

Wyse, DG. (2005). Rate control vs. rhythm control strategies in atrial fibrillation. *Progress in Cardiovascular Diseases* Vol. 48, No. 2, (September-October 2005), pp. 125-138, ISSN 0033-0620

Wyse, DG. & Gersh, BJ. (2004). Atrial fibrillation: a perspective: thinking inside and outside the box. *Circulation* Vol. 109, No. 25, (June 2004), pp. 3089-3095, ISSN 0009-7322

Zhang, GC.; Tsukada, T.; Nakatani, S.; Uematsu, M.; Yasumura, Y.; Tanaka, N.; Masuda, Y.; Miyatake, K. & Yamagishi, M. (1998). Comparison of automatic boundary detection and manual tracking technique in echocardiographic determination of left atrial volume. *Japanese Circulation Journal* Vol. 62, No. 10, (October 1998), pp. 755-759, ISSN 1346-9843

8

Intraoperative Transesophageal Echocardiography for Congenital Heart Disease

Yi-Chia Wang and Chi-Hsiang Huang
National Taiwan University Hospital
Taiwan, R.O.C.

1. Introduction

Transesophageal echocardiography (TEE) has gained its role in perioperative use for congenital heart disease patients, especially with technology improvements in the past decades. It helps with diagnosis confirmation, real-time hemodynamic monitoring, evaluation the successfulness of surgical repair, and surgical planning. The use of intraoperative TEE has major impacts on surgery for congenital heart defects (Randolph et al., 2002). Even with conservative estimates, the financial benefits of TEE in pediatric patients with congenital heart disease are substantial and outweigh its costs (Bettex et al., 2005). In most of the modern cardiac centers, the TEE exam is an essential part of anesthetic management in congenital heart disease surgery.

2. Indication, contraindication, and complications

TEE has proven to be an invaluable tool for patients underwent cardiac surgery and cardiac catheterization for congenital heart disease. More than that, TEE is useful for high risk congenital heart disease patients who will have non-cardiac surgeries. It can help with hemodynamic monitoring, and provide real-time detailed anatomic information. In addition, it can help assess ventricular volume and function, intracardiac shunt, valvular disease, right ventricle (RV) or pulmonary artery (PA) systolic pressure, and pericardial effusions. It is reasonable to use intraoperative TEE routinely in congenital heart surgery (Randolph et al., 2002). According to the "practice guidelines for perioperative TEE", TEE should be used in all adult open heart procedures (Thys et al., 2010). The task force of American Society of Echocardiography also described surgery for congenital heart disease is an indication for performance of TEE (Ayres et al., 2005).

Perioperative TEE exam cannot replace the preoperative diagnostic exam. A thorough imaging study must be performed before the operation. Each imaging study has its limitation. TEE performed before surgical incision may disclose a different diagnosis and even result in cancellation of the operation (Huang et al., 2009).

However, there are some situations that TEE is contraindicated. Patients with unrepaired tracheoesophageal fistula, esophageal obstruction or stricture, perforated hollow organ, or poor airway control should consider transthoracic echocardiography or epicardial echocardiography instead. Besides, patients with history of esophageal surgery, esophageal varices or diverticulum, gastric or esophageal bleeding, oropharyngeal pathology, severe coagulopathy, cervical spine injury or anomaly require extra attention for TEE probe insertion. Although TEE examination is semi-invasive, some people do suffer from complications related to TEE probe insertion (Huang et al., 2007). These include bradycardia due to vagal stimulation, oropharyngeal injury, and esophageal perforation (Kamra et al., 2011). Besides, airway compromise, vascular compression, and dysphagia may be seen after TEE probe insertion. Physicians should respect individual differences and be vigilant to possible complications.

3. Specific defects

3.1 Atrial septal defect

Atrial septal defects (ASD) can be classified into four types: ostium secundum, ostium primum, sinus venosus, and coronary sinus defects (Joffe et al., 2008). The pathophysiological effects of ASD are determined by the defect size and degree of left-to-right shunting. A large defect or unrepaired defect for a long time may lead to right heart volume overload, and subsequent right atrium (RA), RV, and PA dilation.

Ostium secundum ASD is the most commonly encountered ASD. It is located in the central portion of the interatrial septum. Mitral valve prolapse and regurgitation sometimes accompany this defect. With the advancement in treatment, many people now have transcatheter occluder placement instead of surgical patch repair. Mid-esophageal four-chamber and bicaval views delineate the interatrial septum clearly and are used in the evaluation of ASD repair surgery (Figure 1).

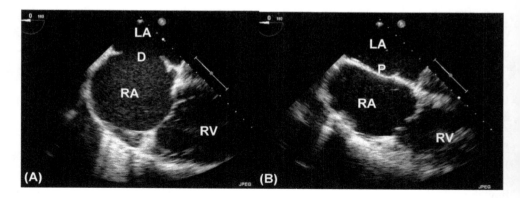

Fig. 1. Secundum atrial septal defect. (A) Preoperative mid-esophageal four-chamber view shows a defect (D) in interatrial septum. (B) The defect is repaired with a patch (P). RA, right atrium; RV, right ventricle; LA, left atrium.

Ostium primum ASD is also known as partial atrioventricular canal defects (see below). It is located in the inferior portion of the interatrial septum. It can be visualized in mid-esophageal four- chamber view (Figure 2). Incomplete formation of the septum primum is sometimes associated with anterior mitral leaflet cleft and regurgitation.

Sinus venosus ASD occurs near the superior vena cava (SVC) or inferior vena cava (IVC) entrance. This kind of defect is often associated with partial anomalous pulmonary venous drainage. After surgical repair, we should look not only for the residual shunt, but also the unobstructed flow in SVC, IVC, and pulmonary veins (Figure 3).

Coronary sinus defects are rare, and result from a communication between the left atrium and coronary sinus. They are commonly associated with a persistent left side SVC.

Preoperative TEE exam should confirm the location, size, shunt magnitude and direction, atrioventricular(AV) valve competence, RA and RV size, associated anomalies, and ventricular function. Post-bypass TEE exam should evaluate the adequacy of surgical repair, valvular competence, and ventricular function.

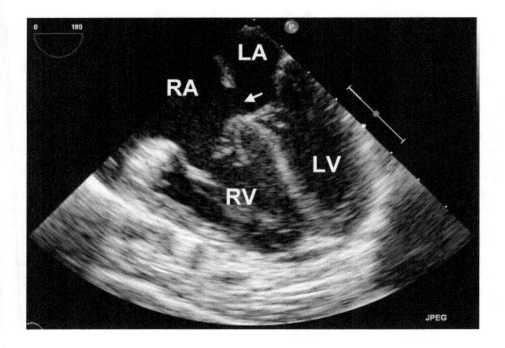

Fig. 2. Mid-esophageal four-chamber view demonstrates a primum atrial septal defect (arrow). RA, right atrium; RV, right ventricle; LA, left atrium; LV, left ventricle.

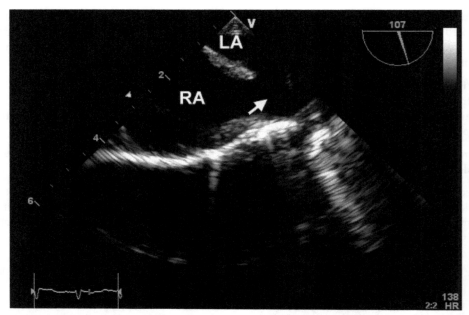

Fig. 3. Modified bicaval view shows a superior sinus venosus atrial septal defect near the superior vena cava and right atrial junction. RA, right atrium; LA, left atrium.

3.2 Ventricular septal defect

Ventricular septal defect (VSD) can be classified by its location to four groups: type I, doubly-committed defects; type II, perimembranous defects; type III, atrioventricular defects; and type IV, muscular defects. Perimembranous and muscular defects can be further subdivided to inlet type, trabecular type, and outlet type according to the extension of the defects (Penny & Vick, 2011). The pathophysiological effects are affected by the size of defect, the systemic and pulmonary vascular resistance, and associated defects such as ASD and patent ductus arteriosus (PDA). The left-to-right shunt can lead to increased left ventricle (LV) volume load, excessive pulmonary blood flow, and decreased systemic cardiac output. A long-standing pulmonary overcirculation may lead to pulmonary hypertension and Eisenmenger's syndrome eventually.

Perimembranous VSDs (Type 2) are confluent with and involve the membranous septum. The defects account for approximately 60-80% of VSDs. Aneurysmal transformation of tricuspid valve may occur and limit the shunt flow. Tricuspid regurgitation (TR) may occur because the tricuspid valve is deformed. Perimembranous outlet defects can associate with aortic cusp prolapse and even aortic insufficiency. Patients with perimembranous defects may develop RV hypertrophy and right ventricular outflow tract (RVOT) narrowing. When the hypertrophied muscular band divides the RV cavity into two chambers, the condition is called double-chambered RV (DCRV) (Figure 4). The outlet septum may be malaligned anteriorly or posteriorly which can possibly result in RVOT or left ventricular outflow tract (LVOT) obstruction respectively.

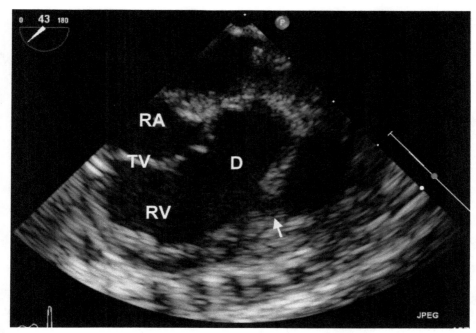

Fig. 4. Perimembranous ventricular septal defect. The right ventricle (RV) inflow-outflow view demonstrates the septal defect (D) and mid-right ventricular obstruction (arrow). RA, right atrium;, TV, tricuspid valve.

Doubly committed, subarterial, or supracristal defects (Type I) are roofed by the arterial valves in fibrous continuity. The defects account for approximately 5% and 30% of VSDs in western and oriental population, respectively. The defects may associate with aortic valve prolapse and aortic insufficiency (Figure 5).

Muscular defects (Type IV) are completely surrounded by a muscular rim. The defects account for about 5-15% of VSDs. Multiple muscular defects can occur (Figure 6). The muscular outlet defects can also associate with aortic cusp prolapse and aortic insufficiency.

Atrioventricular canal or inlet defects (Type III) occur close to the atrioventricular valves in the posterior portion of the ventricular septum. The defects account for approximately 5% of VSDs.

Preoperative TEE exam should confirm the defect location, size, and numbers. Besides, the shunt direction and magnitude, the cardiac chamber size and PA dimension, competence of AV valve, presence of septal malalignment, LVOT or RVOT obstruction, evidence of pulmonary hypertension, and associated cardiac anomalies should be evaluated thoroughly. The velocity of TR jet can be used to calculate PA pressure in the absence of RVOT obstruction. The post-bypass TEE can offer information about the presence of residual shunts or outflow tract obstruction, changes in severity of valvular regurgitation, and ventricular function.

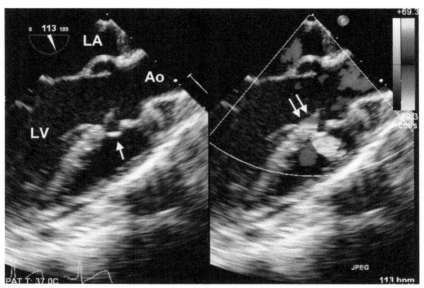

Fig. 5. Doubly-committed ventricular septal defect. Mid-esophageal long-axis view shows the prolapse of aortic cusp (arrow) and the septal defect (double arrow). LA, left atrium; LV, left ventricle; Ao, aorta.

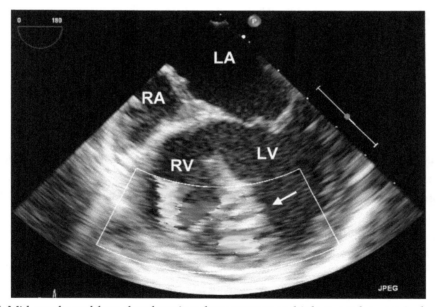

Fig. 6. Mid-esophageal four-chamber view demonstrates multiple muscular ventricular septal defects (arrow). RA, right atrium; RV, right ventricle; LA, left atrium; LV, left ventricle.

3.3 Atrioventricular septal defect

Atrioventricular septal defects (AVSD), also called endocardial cushion defects, are defects involving atrioventricular septum. Normally, mitral valve is attached to a more cephalad position than tricuspid valve. However, in patients with AVSD, their mitral valve and tricuspid valve attach to the same level. There are two types of AVSD, partial AVSD and complete AVSD. In patients with partial AVSD, there is a primum type ASD and anterior mitral leaflet cleft. Though there are usually two orifices for the AV valve, their mitral valve attachment to ventricular septum is not normal, and the leaflet can be thickened, irregular, and dysplasic. Their mitral valve is actually part of the common AV valve and the mitral cleft is a commissure between anterior and posterior bridging leaflets. The attachment of mitral leaflet in the LVOT can cause LVOT obstruction, and poor apposition of the valve can cause mitral regurgitation (MR). Complete AVSD composes single orifice AV valve with deficiency of both atrial and ventricular septum (Figure 7). Rastelli classified this complex into three types according to their different degrees of bridging of superior bridging leaflet, its chordal attachment pattern, and the degree of associative of hypoplasia of the tricuspid anterorsuperior leaflet. The function of common AV valve can be quite variable, ranging from nearly normal function with minimal regurgitation to severely limited dysplastic valve with marked incompetence.

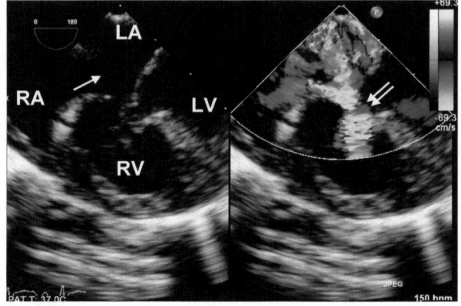

Fig. 7. Complete atrioventricular septal defect. The mid-esophageal four-chamber view shows deficiency of both interatrial (arrow) and interventricular (double arrow) septum.

The pathophysiology of partial AVSD is similar to simple primum ASD. The magnitude of left-to-right shunt is determined by the size of defect and relative ratio of systemic and pulmonary vascular resistance. Mitral cleft can cause significant MR and LV volume overload. The MR can pass the primum ASD and results in LV to RA shunt, RA volume overload, and pulmonary overcirculation. In patients with complete AVSD, the presence of concomitant atrial and ventricular shunting can cause increased shunt flow. Pulmonary hypertension, secondary pulmonary vascular change, and increased pulmonary vascular resistance (PVR) can occur thereafter. The hemodynamic changes are affected by the magnitude and direction of shunt flow. There may be different directions of AV valve regurgitation: LV-to-left atrium (LA), RV-to-RA, LV-to RA, or RV-to-LA.

The mid-esophageal four-chamber view of intraoperative TEE can demonstrate the defect of inferior part of atrial septum. Secundum ASD or patent foramen ovale (PFO) can be present in some patients. The broad-base MR jet not originating from the coaptation may suggest the presence of a cleft mitral valve (Figure 8). Cleft mitral valve may be demonstrated in transgastric basal short-axis view. Besides, the presence of ventricular shunting, sizes of both ventricle, ventricular function, magnitude and direction of AV valve incompetence, degree of AV valve straddling, presence of LVOT obstruction, degree of pulmonary hypertension, and associated cardiac anomalies must be evaluated preoperatively. The postoperative TEE exam should include the evaluation of ventricular function, AV valve competence, and the presence of residual shunt (Cohen et al., 2007). Because valvular regurgitation is quite pressure and load dependent, it is important that we take patient's volume status and cardiac contractility into consideration when comparing preoperative and postoperative regurgitation severity. If prosthetic valve is replaced, it is important to check the function of prosthetic valve and the presence of paravalvular leak.

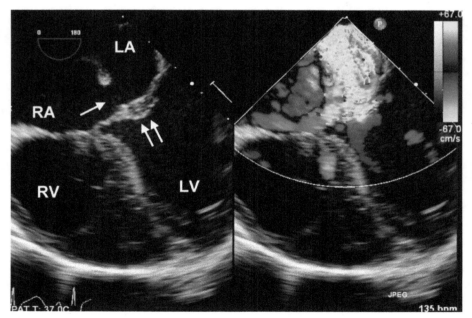

Fig. 8. Partial atrioventricular septal defect. The mid-esophageal four-chamber view demonstrates a primum atrial septal defect (atrial) and mitral cleft (double arrow) with severe mitral regurgitation.

3.4 Patent ductus arteriosus and aortopulmonary window

PDA is a postnatal communication between the main pulmonary trunk and descending thoracic aorta due to persistent patency of fetal ductus arteriosus (Schneider & Moore, 2006). Shunt flow is determined by diameter of PDA and the pressure gradient. The preoperative TEE can demonstrate the shunt flow in the ascending aorta short-axis view (Figure 9). The size of left-side chambers, ventricular function, valvular regurgitation, degree of pulmonary hypertension, and associated cardiac anomalies must also be evaluated. The postoperative TEE exam can be used to detect the presence of residual ductal flow.

Aortopulmonary defect, also known as aortopulmonary (AP) window, is a defect between ascending aorta and pulmonary artery. Without treatment, pulmonary system will be overloaded due to left to right shunt, and eventually develop pulmonary vascular occlusive disease. A significant portion of the patients have other associated cardiac anomalies. Preoperative TEE can detect a shunt between ascending aorta and PA (Figure 10). Evidence of pulmonary hypertension, ventricular function and size, defect size and shunt pressure gradient can be measured by intraoperative TEE. Surgical treatment usually involves aorta incision, defect visualization, and a patch is sutured to close the defect over the aortic side. The post-repair TEE exam should detect the presence of residual shunt, valvular competence, and ventricular function.

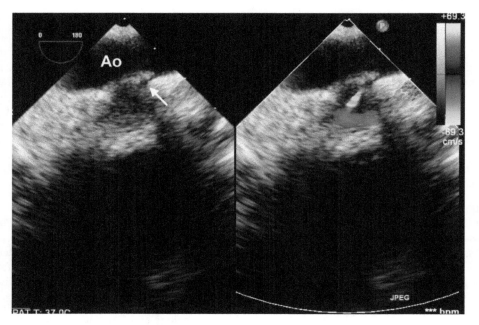

Fig. 9. The upper esophageal aortic arch long-axis view demonstrates the patent ductus arteriosus (arrow) connecting aortic arch and left pulmonary artery. Ao, aorta.

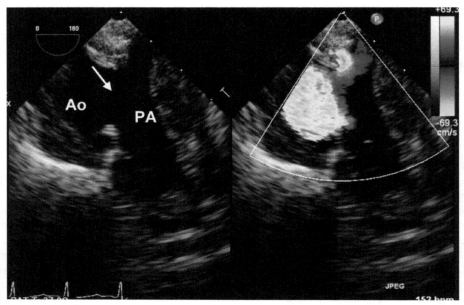

Fig. 10. Aortopulmonary window as a defect (arrow) between ascending aorta and main pulmonary artery. Ao, aorta; PA, pulmonary artery.

3.5 Truncus arteriosus

Truncus arteriosus is caused by failure of truncal ridge and aortopulmonary septum to develop, forming aorta and PA. There is a single great vessel arising from a common semilunar valve, and a VSD. The truncal valve can have variable cusps, and valvular incompetence is not uncommon. Further classification is dependent on the existence of truncal septum, and the take-off position of pulmonary arteries. The VSD is caused by failure of conal septum to develop and rotate. It is usually large, non-restrictive, with superior border adjacent to truncal valve. PA is usually of normal size, but stenosis at origin site or diffuse hypoplasia may happen. Other common concurrent cardiac defects include right aortic arch, PDA, persistent left-sided SVC, ASD, and anomalous subclaivan artery.

Surgical repair encompasses separation of branched PA from truncus vessel, establishment of RV-PA continuity by RVOT reconstruction or RV-PA conduit, VSD closure, and repair of associated anomalies. Due to variable coronary anatomy, separation of PA from truncal vessel should be done with care. Mild to moderate truncal valve regurgitation is often tolerated, and will improve over time. However, severe regurgitation is a poor indicator for long term survival. If the truncal valve is severely incompetent, valve replacement should be considered.

Intraoperative TEE should focus on truncal valve morphology and function, anatomy of the main and branched pulmonary arteries, size and position of the intracardiac shunting, AV valve competence, ventricular function and the associated cardiac abnormalities (Figure 11).

After repair, truncal valve function, residual intracardiac shunt and RVOT patency can be examined with color Doppler. Monitoring of ventricular function is important, because coronary artery may be compromised during pulmonary artery resection, RV-PA conduit reconstruction, and reimplantation of coronary arteries. Pulmonary hypertensive crisis and low cardiac output are potential threats for patients undergoing repair. RV function and severity of TR demonstrated in TEE exam can give anesthesiologist a guide for patient management.

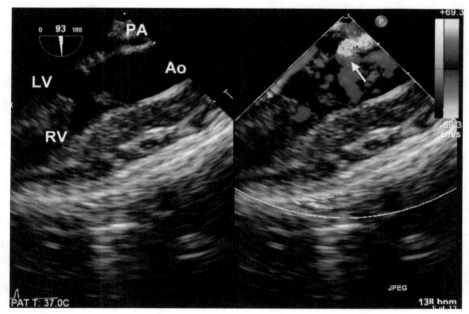

Fig. 11. The mid-esophageal long-axis view shows a truncal vessel overrides the left ventricle (LV) and right ventricle (RV) and gives rise to aorta and pulmonary artery (arrow). Ao, aorta; PA, pulmonary artery.

3.6 Coarctation of aorta and interrupted aortic arch

Coarctation of aorta (CoA) is characterized by narrowing of aortic lumen due to thickening or infolding of aortic media (Rosenthal, 2005). Interrupted aortic arch (IAA), on the other hand, is complete discontinuity between two parts of aortic arch. These lesions lie closely to PDA or ligament arterioum. In patients with CoA, the defect can be isolated, or associated with VSD or other complex cardiac disease. The LV afterload is increased in patients with CoA. The site and extent of the stenosis may be seen in upper esophageal level during TEE exam (Figure 12). However, preoperative TEE exam can offer valuable information for other associated anomalies, such as biscupid aortic valve, Shone's complex, and VSD. Surgical treatment includes resection of stenotic area with end-to-end anastomosis, extended resection with primary anastomosis, subclavian flap aortoplasty, and patch augmentation. Some patients have balloon angioplasty and stent insertion in intervention units. Postoperative TEE gives a direct evidence of anatomic site patency and LV function.

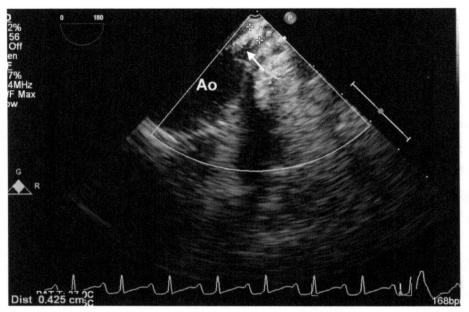

Fig. 12. Upper esophageal aortic arch long-axis view shows coarctation of aorta (arrow). Ao, aorta.

IAA is classified by its interruption location into three types: type A, interruption is distal to left subclavian artery; type B, interruption is between left subclavian artery and left common carotid artery; and type C, interruption is proximal to left carotid artery. The arterial circulation proximal to the interruption is supplied by the LV output. The RV output supplies the arterial circulation distal to the interruption via the ductus arteriosus. Patients usually have PDA, VSD, and aortic valve abnormalities. The VSD is usually conoventricular type with a posterior conal septum malalignment, which causes LVOT obstruction at either subvalvular or valvular level.

Preoperative TEE can be used to evaluate the morphology of aortic arch and PDA. Other coexisting defects should be carefully explored. Size of LVOT and aortic valve should be measured. Failure to detect LVOT obstruction is likely to result in persistent heart failure postoperatively. Surgical treatment for IAA is more complex than simple CoA. Current favorable approach is one-stage repair of interruption, and total correction of intracardiac abnormalities. However, if LVOT obstruction prohibited one-stage correction, modified Norwood operation such as Damus-Kaye-Stansel connection with atrial septectomy may be needed. Postbyapss TEE exam should survey for anastomotic stenosis, aortic or subaortic obstruction, residual atrial or ventricular shunts, and signs of pulmonary hypertension.

3.7 Anomalous pulmonary venous return

Partial or total anomalous pulmonary venous return (PAPVR/TAPVR) indicates that some or all of the pulmonary veins enter systemic venous circulation instead of LA. According to the connection site of pulmonary veins, anomalous pulmonary venous return (APVR) can be classified as supracardiac type, cardiac type, infracardiac type, and mixed type. In supracardiac type APVR, confluence of pulmonary veins unites to an ascending vertical vein and joins the innominate vein, and then drains into SVC and RA. Sometimes the vertical vein bypasses the innominate vein and joins SVC directly. The connection site between vertical vein and innominate vein or SVC is prone for pulmonary venous obstruction. In patients with cardiac type APVR, the pulmonary vein confluence drains into the coronary sinus, and then to the RA. Some of the patients will have pulmonary veins going directly to RA. In the infracardiac type, the pulmonary vein confluence drains into a descending vertical vein, goes down across diaphragm to portal vein or hepatic vein, and then comes back to RA with IVC.

The pathophysiology is similar to that of ASD in patients with PAPVR. The degree of shunt is determined by the numbers of anomalous pulmonary venous connections. In TAPVR, all of the pulmonary veins drain into RA and there is no pulmonary venous return in LA. Blood in LA is derived from PFO or ASD, which is mixed deoxygenated blood, therefore the patients are cyanotic. In patients with small size or restrictive ASD, the systemic circulation will decrease significantly. In patients with large or nonrestrictive ASD, the magnitude of shunt is determined by the relative ratio of PVR and systemic vascular resistance (SVR).

The pulmonary veins are in the posterior portion of the heart, which makes TEE a valuable tool for optimal imaging and Doppler examination. However, proper probe size should be considered to avoid pulmonary veins compression by probe insertion. PAPVR should be suspected whenever a sinus venous ASD is present. The distinguishable TEE feature of TAPVR includes absence of pulmonary venous connection to LA, identification of alternate pulmonary venous drainage site, and RV overload (Figure 13). The presence of pulmonary venous obstruction, pulmonary hypertension and associated cardiac anomalies must be evaluated. The post-repair TEE exam should check the ventricular and valvular function, signs of pulmonary hypertension, and presence of pulmonary venous obstruction.

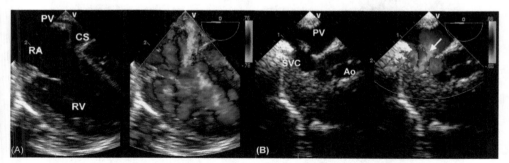

Fig. 13. Anomalous pulmonary venous return. (A) Cardiac type: the modified mid-esophageal four-chamber view demonstrates the drainage of pulmonary vein (PV) into coronary sinus (CS) and then right atrium (RA). (B) Supracardiac type: the modified mid-esophageal five-chamber view shows the dainage of PV into superior vena cava (SVC) (arrow). RV, right ventricle; Ao, aorta.

3.8 Tetralogy of fallot

Tetralogy of Fallot (TOF) consists of VSD, overriding aorta, RVOT obstruction, and RV hypertrophy. It can be associated with right aortic arch, additional VSDs, absence of the pulmonic valve, coronary artery anomalies, systemic venous anomalies, AP window, and LVOT obstruction. Surgery involves VSD closure and repair or reconstruction of RVOT (Shinebourne et al., 2006).

The pathophysiological changes in patients with TOF are related to the shunt flow across a large VSD and the degree of RVOT obstruction. RV pressure is increased due to large VSD flow and RVOT obstruction. When the RV pressure is greater than systemic pressure, a right-to-left shunt and arterial desaturation will ensue. There may be little or no right-to-left shunt if the RVOT obstruction is not severe. The common associated cardiac anomalies include right-sided aortic arch in 25%, ASD in 10%, and coronary anomalies in 10% of patients with TOF.

Preoperative TEE exam can evaluate the degree of RV hypertrophy and aortic overriding, the site and severity of RVOT obstruction, size and location of VSD, direction and magnitude of shunt flow, ventricular and valvular function, morphology of pulmonary arteries, and associated cardiac lesions such as ASD. Overriding aorta and anterior malalignment of outlet septum can be best seen in mid-esophageal aortic valve long-axis view (Figure 14). RVOT obstruction and shunt across VSD can be evaluated in mid-esophageal RV inflow-outflow view (Figure 15). Valvular and supravalvular pulmonary stenosis can be demonstrated in upper-esophageal aortic short-axis view. Post-repair TEE evaluation should include the presence and degree of residual RVOT obstruction, residual intracardiac shunt, peripheral pulmonary stenosis, aortic and pulmonary regurgitation, and ventricular function.

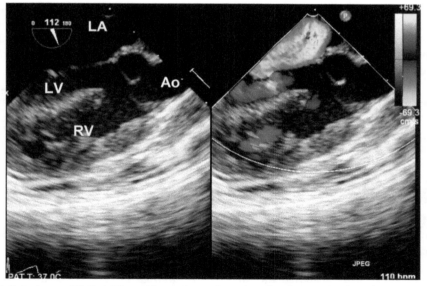

Fig. 14. Tetralogy of Fallot. The mid-esophageal aortic valve long-axis view demonstrates the overriding of aorta. LA, left atrium; LV, left ventricle; RV, right ventricle; Ao, aorta.

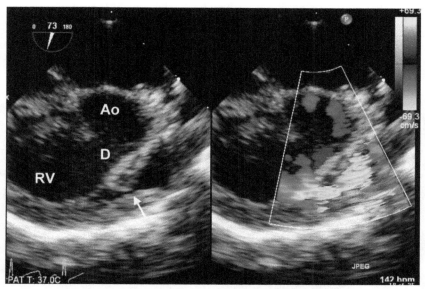

Fig. 15. Tetralogy of Fallot. The right ventricle (RV) inflow-outflow view shows a ventricular septal defect (D) and infundibular pulmonary stenosis (arrow). Ao, aorta.

3.9 Ebstein's anomaly

Ebstein's anomaly is characterized by abnormal attachment of septal and posterior tricuspid leaflets in the RV, away from normal tricuspid annulus position. The anterior leaflet is normally attached at annulus, but morphologically enlarged, "sail-like", and tethered to RV wall. The anterior leaflet may functionally obstruct the RVOT. Because tricuspid valve orifice is displaced downward to RV cavity at the junction of the inlet and trabecular components, the proximal portion of the RV is functionally integrated into RA, termed atrialized RV. The severity of hemodynamic compromise is related to the downward displacement of the leaflets, the degree of outflow tract obstruction and valvular regurgitation, the severity of myocardial dysfunction, and other concomitant cardiac abnormalities. RV output is decreased by decreased RV volume and varying degrees of RVOT obstruction. The most commonly accompanied disease is secundum type ASD or PFO. Cyanosis will occur if there is a large right-to-left shunt. Clinical presentation varied extremely from normal tricuspid function found incidentally on autopsy to severe cyanosis, compromised cardiac function, and fetal death. Appropriate surgical intervention depends on the age at presentation and associated anomalies. Tricuspid valve is either repaired or replaced depending on the extent of atrialized ventricle and morphology of tricuspid valve. Single ventricle repair may be performed in patients with poor RV condition.

Considering the variety of the disease entity and different surgical approaches, intraoperative TEE has a significant role in preoperative evaluation and decision making. In mid-esophageal four-chamber view, we can calculate the displacement index, which is the apical displacement of tricuspid valve septal leaflet in millimeters indexed to body surface area. A displacement index more than $8mm/m^2$ is a sensitive predictor of Ebstein's anomaly

(Oechslin et al. 2000). The preoperative TEE evaluation should include the RA dimension, size and shunt magnitude of ASD, the morphology of tricuspid leaflets, the severity of TR, the presence of RVOT obstruction, ventricular function, and associated cardiac anomalies (Figure 16). Postoperatively, we should evaluate tricuspid valve function, residual intracardiac shunting, residual RVOT obstruction, and RV dysfunction.

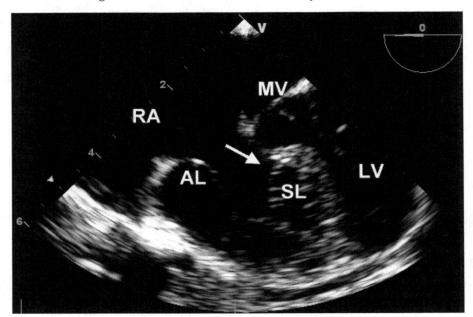

Fig. 16. Ebstein's anomaly. The mid-esophageal four-chamber view demonstrates the "sail-like" anterior leaflet (AL) of tricuspid valve and downward attachment (arrow) of septal leaflet (SL) of tricuspid valve. RA, right atrium; LV, left ventricle; MV, mitral valve.

3.10 Transposition of great arteries / congenitally corrected transposition of great arteries

Dextro-transposition of great arteries (d-TGA) stands for 5-7% in congenital heart disease. It is characterized by concordance of the AV connection and discordance of the ventriculoarterial (VA) connection. Without treatment, 30% of patients will die in one week, 50% of patients will die in one month, and 90% of patients will die in one year. Balloon atrial septostomy and prostaglandin E1 for PDA patency are usually given for flow communication. Preoperative TEE exam should include the assessment of the AV and VA connections, outflow tract obstruction, systemic to pulmonary communications, ventricular size and function, and the associated cardiac pathology (Figure 17).

Surgical treatment for d-TGA has changed significantly through the years. Before mid 1980, the favored approach for infants with d-TGA is atrial switch procedure (Mustard or Senning operation). Surgeons will redirect the blood flow from SVC and IVC through mitral valve, then to LV. The heart will pump the blood from LV to PA. Pulmonary vein flow will be directed to RV, aorta, and systemic circulation. This changes the parallel, non-communicating circulation to serial connection with oxygenation. The intraoperative study mainly involves an assessment of systemic and pulmonary venous pathways. We should look for obstruction of systemic and pulmonary venous return, baffle leak, and ventricular function. Though atrial switch operation corrects hemodynamic abnormalities, it does not correct anatomical imperfections. Later complications include systemic RV failure, baffle obstruction, and arrhythmia.

Arterial switch operation, the Jatene procedure, has been performed for anatomical repair since 1980s (Skinner et al., 2008). The great arteries are transected above the sinus valsalva and anastomosed to their appropriate ventricular outflows. Coronary arteries are translocated to the systemic outflow. Perioperative TEE should evaluate the size and flow of two neo-arteries, and check for any valvular stenosis or regurgitation. Because coronary arteries are relocated, TEE becomes an important tool for segmental and global function evaluation, thus providing indirect evidence of coronary perfusion.

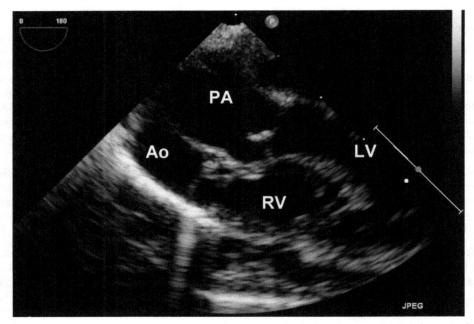

Fig. 17. Transposition of great arteries. The pulmonary artery (PA) arises from left ventricle (LV) and the aorta (Ao) arises from right ventricle (RV).

Levo-transposition of great arteries (l-TGA), also commonly referred to as congenitally corrected transposition of the great arteries (ccTGA), is an acyanotic congenital heart disease. In segmental analysis, this condition is described as AV discordance and VA discordance, with aorta anterior and to the left of the PA. RV serves as the systemic ventricle. Although the physiology of blood flow is correct, systemic RV may develop failure progressively.

Double switch operation may be performed for patients with l-TGA. It is a combination of atrial switch operation and arterial switch operation. The preoperative TEE exam should evaluate the relationship of great arteries, presence of outflow tract obstruction, ventricular and valvular function, and associated intracardiac anomalies. The post-repair TEE exam should focus on the systemic and pulmonary venous return pathway, ventricular and valvular function, and anatomy of outflow tract and neo-great arteries.

3.11 Double outlet right ventricle

The key feature of double outlet right ventricle (DORV) is the two great arteries arising primarily from RV. For each artery, RV should contribute more than 50% of it blood flow. There are four types of VSD in DORV patients: subaortic VSD, subpulmonary VSD, doubly committed VSD, and remote VSD. DORV with subaortic VSD is the most common variety in DORV. The conal septum here usually deviates anterior and leftward, and sometimes causes subpulmonary or pulmonary valve stenosis. If there is no pulmonary stenosis, pulmonary blood flow is determined by the relationship of SVR and PVR. If the VSD is subaortic and pulmonary stenosis exists, the presentation is similar to TOF. The degree of cyanosis is dependent on the severity of pulmonary flow obstruction.

DORV with subpulmonary VSD is caused by malalignment of conal septum, which should be differentiated from pure subpulmonary VSD. The conal septum is deviated to posterior and right, sometime causing subaortic narrowing. The Taussig-Bing malformation is a special variant of DORV with subpulmonary VSD, side by side great arteries, aorta at right side, and bilateral subarterial conus. The physiology of this variant is similar to d-TGA. Cyanosis is usually caused by inadequate mixing of systemic and pulmonary circulation, and improved atrial or ductal mixing by emergent balloon atrial septostomy and prostaglandin E1 may be needed.

In DORV with doubly committed VSD, conal septum is deficient, and VSD is usually nonrestrictive. The prevalence is rare, and the hemodynamic is determined by out flow tract obstructions. In DORV with remote VSD or noncommitted VSD, the defects can be within muscular septum or AV canal septum. Because the distance of VSD and semilunar valves are far, surgical management is sometimes restricted.

Different anatomical arrangements have impacts on hemodynamic presentation, and influence the surgical planning (Lancour-Gayet, 2008). In addition to confirming diagnosis, preoperative TEE should provide information that help to determine a suitable surgical procedure. The size and relative position of VSD to great artery locations should be evaluated by preoperative TEE. Color Doppler gives information of outflow tract obstruction. The presence of pulmonary stenosis or aortic stenosis, either valvular or subvalvular, can be imaged in multiple views. The relative size of both ventricles, the presence of AV valve straddling, the pulmonary valve to tricuspid valve distance, and presence of other associated cardiac anomalies should all be evaluated by preoperative TEE (Figure 18).

In most cases, the goal of surgery is to complete biventricular repair and restore normal circulation. Surgeons will establish unobstructed LV to aorta continuity, establish adequate RV to PA continuity, and repair associated lesions. Some patients with DORV and subpulmonary VSD are repaired with arterial switch operation after baffling the LV to PA through VSD. Occasionally, in patients with unbalanced ventricle or other associated anomalies, two-ventricle repair is not feasible and operation toward single ventricle physiology is needed.

Postoperative complications generally fall into four groups: LV failure, RV failure, arrhythmia, and residual shunts. Because LV flow is baffled through VSD to great artery, obstruction occurs with poor configuration of the patch or insufficient enlarged VSD size. It is especially difficult in DORV with remote VSD. Aortic insufficiency may occur due to surgical damage. Residual RVOT obstruction can occur whether the repair acquired infundibulotomy, outflow tract patch, or some form of RV to PA conduit. Intracardiac baffle may compromise RVOT flow, especially in DORV with subpulmonary VSD, because the VSD is very close to pulmonary orifice and infundibular septal band. Tricuspid insufficiency may happen if chordae resection and reattachment is needed to accommodate baffle implantation. After arterial switch operation, neo-PA or branched PA obstruction should be carefully surveyed. Residual shunt may be caused by incomplete VSD repair, baffle detachment, and unrecognized multiple VSDs. It is prudent to carefully evaluate the repair by TEE before leaving operation room.

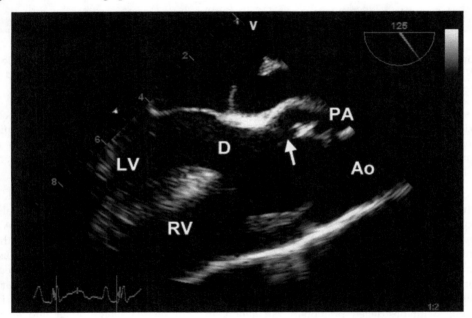

Fig. 18. Double-outlet right ventricle. The mid-esophageal long-axis view demonstrates both aorta (Ao) and pulmonary artery (PA) arises from right ventricle (RV) and the presence of pulmonary stenosis (arrow) and ventricular septal defect (D). LV, left ventricle; RV, right ventricle.

3.12 Single ventricular physiology

The functionally univentricular circulation, or single-ventricle physiology, is a heterogenous group of cardiac abnormalities. In most patients, there is hypoplasia of either the RV or LV which is unable to maintain a pulmonary or systemic circulation independently (Khairy et al., 2007). This anatomical category includes hypoplastic left heart syndrome, tricuspid atresia, and double-inlet LV (Figure 19). Two-ventricular repair may not be feasible in some complex congenital heart disease even with balanced ventricles, such as malpositioned or straddling AV valve, or DORV with a remote VSD, and single ventricle management strategy must be undertaken.

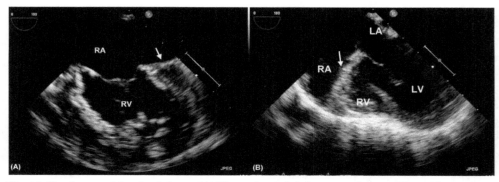

Fig. 19. Single ventricle physiology. (A) Hypoplastic left heart syndrome. The mid-esophageal short-axis view shows the mitral atresia (arrow) and hypoplasia of left ventricle (LV). (B) Tricuspid atresia. The mid-esophageal short-axis view demonstrates the tricuspid atresia (arrow) and hypoplasia of right ventricle (RV). RA, right atrium.

In single ventricle anatomy, the functional ventricle provides a common mixing chamber, and must pump both the systemic and pulmonary circulations, which easily lead to volume overload, cyanosis, or congestive heart failure. This pathophysiology encompasses a complex group of diseases. The presence of systemic and pulmonary outflow tract obstruction both contribute to the clinical manifestation.

Current surgical management of single ventricle is divided into 3 stages. Stage I operation technique is dependent on patients' status. Surgical palliation is to achieve following goals: unobstructive systemic blood flow, balanced and limited pulmonary blood flow, minimal AV valve regurgitation, nondistorted pulmonary arteries, and unrestricted return of blood to the ventricle. If pulmonary flow is unrestricted, pulmonary banding is done to minimize ventricular overload and avoid pulmonary hypertension. If systemic obstruction is noted, Norwood operation or Damus-Kaye-Stansel palliation is used. A systemic to pulmonary shunt, such as Blalock-Taussig (B-T) shunt is placed to provide pulmonary blood flow in patients with obstructed pulmonary circulation. In addition, AV valve repair and atrial septostomy may be needed according to patients' condition. The preoperative TEE exam includes the evaluation of AV and VA connections, AV valve morphology and function, degree of outflow tract obstruction, size and morphology of ventricles, and associated cardiac anomalies. The postoperative TEE exam should focus on the presence of systemic outflow tract obstruction, AV valve function, status of pulmonary blood flow and ventricular function.

Stage II operation mainly aims to connect SVC to PA and eliminate or restrict other sources for pulmonary blood flow. Bidirectional Glenn shunt and hemi-Fontan anastomosis are representatives. Bidirectional Glenn shunt is built from SVC to PA. After the operation, the driving force to pulmonary circulation is SVC pressure. Part of the left to right shunt is removed, and thus relieving the volume load from single ventricle. Perioperative TEE exam includes the evaluation of the anastomosis site, PA morphology,AV valve function, and ventricular function.

Current approach for stage III operation is Fontan operation or total cavopulmonary connection. Intracardiac lateral tunnel or extracardiac conduit may be used to create cavopulmonary connection. In this stage, pulmonary flow is dependent on systemic venous pressure, and all the pulmonary flow is effective. Fontan fenestration is sometimes provided to offer a source to systemic circulation that is not dependent on passing through pulmonary circulation. The perioperative TEE exam includes evaluation of the patency of cavopulmonary connection, AV valve function, size and flow of fenestration, and ventricular function (Figure 20).

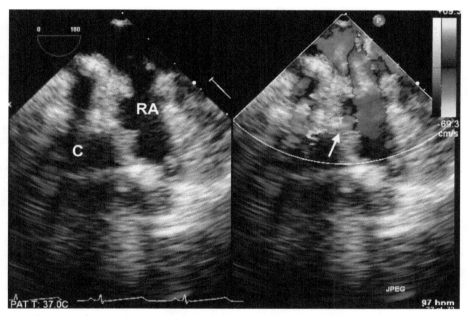

Fig. 20. There is a fenestration with shunt flow (arrow) between the extracardiac conduit (C) and right atrium (RA) after total cavopulmonary connection in a patient with tricuspid atresia.

4. Conclusion

Congenital heart disease is a complex disease entity of various severities. Intraoperative TEE offers valuable information about patients' anatomy and pathophysiology. In addition to diagnosis confirmation, TEE is a useful guide for surgical planning and anesthetic management. Intraoperative assessment by TEE images may be difficult due to complicated pathological presentations. A thorough understanding of anatomy, pathophysiology, and surgical procedure of congenital heart disease is required for interpretation of intraoperative TEE.

5. References

Ayres, NA., Miller-Hance, W., Fyfe DA, et al.(2005) Indications and guidelines for performance of transesophageal echocardiography in the patient with pediatric acquired or congenital heart disease. A report from the task force of the pediatric council of the American society of echocardiography. *Journal of American Society of Echocardiography*, Vol.18, No.1, pp. 91-98.

Bettex, DA., Pretre, R., Jenni, R., et al.(2005) Cost-effectiveness of routine intraoperative transesophageal echocardiography in pediatric cardiac surgery: a 10-year experience. *Anesthesia & Analgesia*, Vol.100, No.5, pp. 1271-1275.

Cohen, GA. & Stevenson, JG. (2007) Intraoperative echocardioraphy for atrioventricular canal: decision-making for surgeons. *Seminars in Thoracic and Cardiovascular Syrgery: Pediatric Cardiac Surgery Annual*, Vol.10, No.1, pp. 47-50.

Huang, CH., Lu, CW., Lin, TY., et al. (2007) Complications of intraoperative transesophageal echocardiography in adult cardiac patients—experience of two institutions in Taiwan. *Journal of the Formosan Medical Association*, Vol.106, No.1, pp. 92-95.

Huang, HH., Lin, PL., Chao, IF., Chao, A. & Huang, CH. (2009) Misdiagnosed right atrial tumor identified by intraoperative transesophageal echocardiography. *Cardiology Journal*, Vol.16, No.2, pp. 175-176.

Joffe, DC., Rivo, J., Oxorn, DC. (2008) Coronary sinus atrial septal defect. *Anesthesia & Analgesia*, Vol.107, No.4, pp. 1163-1165.

Kamra, K., Russell, I., Miller-Hance, WC. (2011) Role of transesophageal echocardiography in the management of pediatric patients with congenital heart disease. *Paediatric Anaesthesia*, Vol.21, No.5, pp. 479-493.

Khairy, P., Poirier, N., Mercier, LA. (2007) Univentricular heart. *Circulation*, Vol.115, No.6, pp. 800-812.

Lacour-Gayet, F. (2008) Intracardiac repair of double outlet right ventricle. *Seminars in Thoracic and Cardiovascular Syrgery: Pediatric Cardiac Surgery Annual*, Vol.11, No.1, pp. 39-43.

Oechslin, E., Buchholz, S., Jenni, R. (2000) Ebstein's anomaly in adults: Doppler-echocardiographic evaluation. *The Thoracic & Cardiovascular Surgeon*, Vol.48, No.4, pp. 209-213.

Penny, DJ. & Vick, GW. (2011) Ventricular septal defect. *Lancet*, Vol.377, No.9771, pp. 1103-1112.

Randolph, GR., Hagler, DJ., Connolly, HM., et al.(2002) Intraoperative transesophageal echocardiography during surgery for congenital heart defects. *Journal of Thoracic & Cardiovascular Surgery*, Vol.124, No.6, pp. 1176-1182.

Rosenthal, E. (2005) Coarctation of aorta from fetus to adult: curable condition of life long disease process? *Heart*, Vol.91, No.11, pp. 1495-1502.

Schneider,DJ., & Moore, JW. (2006) Patent ductus arteriosus. *Circulation*, Vol.114, No.17, pp. 1873-1882.

Shinebourne, EA., Babu-Narayan, SV., Carvalho, JS. (2006) Tetralogy of Fallot: from fetus to adult. *Heart*, Vol.92, No.9, pp. 1353-1359.

Skinner, J., Hornung, T., Rumball, E. (2008) Transposition of the great arteries: from fetus to adult. *Heart*, Vol.94, No.9, pp. 1227-1235.

Thys, DM., Abel, MD., Brooker, RF., et al.(2010) Practice guidelines for perioperative transesophageal echocardiography. An updated report by the American society of anesthesiologistsand the society of cardiovascular anesthesiologists task force on transesophageal echocardiography. *Anesthesiology*, Vol.112, No.5, pp. 1084-1096.

Part 3

Echocardiography in Special Disease

9

Cardiac Tumors

Maryam Moshkani Farahani
Department of Echocardiography, Faculty of Medicine,
Baqiyatallah University of Medical Sciences,
Molla Sadra Avenue, Tehran
Iran

1. Introduction

Cardiac tumors are among important group of cardiovascular diseases. Early diagnosis is necessary for the best management of the tumors. There are several imaging modalities available for cardiac tumors for diagnosis including echocardiography (transthoracic echocardiography, transesophageal echocardiography, 3 dimensional echocardiography) magnetic resonance imaging (MRI) and CT scan. However, echocardiography remains the best available noninvasive tool for the diagnosis of cardiac masses, while CT and MRI provide more information about the texture and extension of tumor.

Echocardiography provides useful information about the size, texture, location, extension of tumors, hemodynamic effects on heart such as stenosis.

Cardiac tumors can be found incidentally such as myxoma or left atrial thrombus in a patient with mitral stenosis. There is also different clinical presentation for cardiac masses such as constitutional symptoms, embolic events, fever etc.

Two groups of tumors can involve the heart: primary and secondary tumors. Primary tumors are rare with a prevalence of 0.001 to 0.03 percent in autopsies (1).The majority of primary tumors are benign such as myxoma, the most common form of primary tumors, responsible for half of these tumors (2). One fourth of cardiac tumors are malignant, and sarcomas with primary cardiac lymphomas are the most common malignant primary cardiac tumors (3).

Malignant primary cardiac tumors include: angiosarcoma, rhabdomyosarcoma, osteosarcoma, myxosarcoma, fibrosarcoma and synovial sarcoma. Various sarcomas and lymphomas are the most common primary malignant cardiac tumors (4, 5).

Metastatic tumors are 20 to 40 times more common than primary malignant ones with prevalence of 6% in post-mortem autopsies in malignant diseases (6). The most common tumors that metastasize to heart are from lung, breast, kidney, and liver; and among tumor variety, lymphoma, melanoma and osteogenic sarcoma (2).

Malignant tumors can metastasize to heart via hematogenous spread from inferior vena cava such as renal and hepatic tumors or via metastatic formation by systemic tumors such as malignant melanoma, lymphomas, leukaemias and sarcomas. Lymphatics and direct invasion from adjacent organs such as lung and breast cancers or mediastinal lymphomas is another way of spread (7, 6).

2. Benign primary cardiac tumors

2.1 Myxoma

Three quarters of all primary cardiac tumors are benign and half of them are myxomas. These tumors occur mostly in third decade or later. Myxomas can occur as an isolated tumor in left atrium (the most common site of this tumor)[figure 1] or as familial form (Carney syndrome) which is associated with other manifestations. Most frequently it occurs in left atrium, then in right atrium, right ventricle and left ventricle; it can infrequently involve the valves. It is mostly attached to fossa ovalis via its stalk.

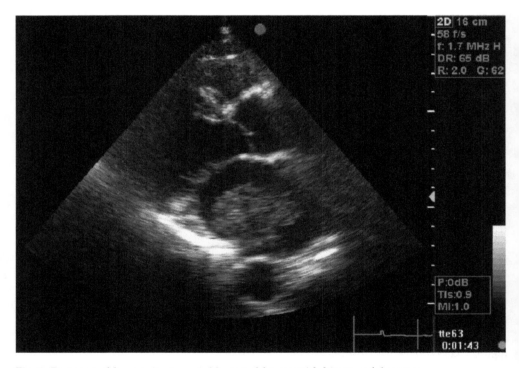

Fig. 1. Parasternal long axis view. A 38 year old man with history of dyspnea. Echocardiography revealed left atrial mass. He underwent cardiac surgery and pathology showed myxoma.

Myxoma has different clinical presentations. These include constitutional symptoms such as fever, weight loss, embolic events and symptoms of valvular obstruction such as the symptoms of mitral valve stenosis (figure 2).

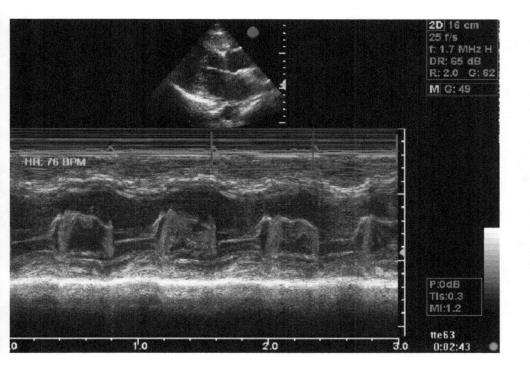

Fig. 2. A 38 year old man with history of dyspnea. Myxoma can protrude through mitral valve and in M-mode mitral stenosis can be visualized as seen in this Echocardiograph.

It has also different shapes as rounded or polypoid with narrow stalk and attachment to interatrial septum or fossa ovalis. The mass is mostly homogenous; however, small scattered area of calcification may be seen. Mobile particles of this tumor describe and predict its tendency for embolic events (8).

Echocardiography provides useful information about the location, size, extension and texture of this tumor, and one should be careful not to miss the multiple myxomas that could be found in other chambers.

Definite treatment for myxoma is total excision of the mass. Follow up echocardiography to rule out recurrence is recommended.

2.2 Papillary fibroelastoma

Papillary fibroelastoma is a rare, primary benign cardiac tumor that is most frequently found in the cardiac valves (9). It is the third primary cardiac tumor after myxoma and lipoma. These tumors are mostly found incidentally on post mortem. However, because of high tendency for systemic emboli, prompt diagnosis and management is necessary. Other rare presentations such as sudden death have been reported (10-12).

Papillary fibroelastoma represents 7.9% of benign primary cardiac tumor in adults (9). Approximately 90% of primary fibroelastomas arise from valves on ventricular side of pulmonary and aortic valve and atrial side of mitral and tricuspid valve (13-14). Aortic or mitral valves are mostly affected (15-16). The tricuspid valve is most affected in children; however, mitral and aortic valves are mostly affected in adults (17). Echocardiography remains the main tool for detection of this tumor. Because of involvement of cardiac valves other diagnosis such as infective endocarditis, degenerative changes and 0Lamble's excrescences should be kept in mind. Typical echocardiographic features include round, oval or irregular appearance, with a homogenous texture with small stalk (18). Surgical removal is indicated for large mobile tumors.

2.3 Rhabdomyoma

It is the most frequent cardiac tumor of childhood (about 60% of cardiac tumors) which is frequently found by fetal echocardiography (8). This tumor occurs in both ventricles equally with intramural involvement; however, atrioventricular valves involvement is also seen. This tumor may regress spontaneously.

2.4 Lipoma

It is a benign cardiac tumor that is asymptomatic in many patients (3). CT scan or MRI can easily define the tissue characteristic of fat and make an accurate diagnosis.

2.5 Hemangioma

It is a benign vascular tumor which occurs equally in left and right ventricles, and in right atrium. When tumor is resectable, total excision is recommended. Other benign cardiac tumors include cardiac paraganglioma (8) and fibroma.

3. Malignant primary cardiac tumors

Sarcomas are the most common primary malignant tumors and consist of 95% of cases. Any part of heart can be affected and rapid progression of disease is the usual clinical course of this tumor (8).

3.1 Angiosarcoma

Angiosarcoma is the most common primary malignant cardiac tumor (7). Men are involved more than female with a ratio of 2:1. Its usual location is right atrium and interatrial septum with involvement of pericardium and pericardial effusion [figure 3] (8). Other forms of sarcoma can occur in the left side of the heart and resemble the presentation of myxoma. It has a poor prognosis.

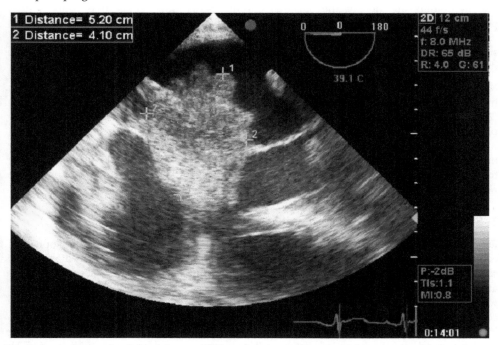

Fig. 3. Large tumor in right atrium with invasion toward interatrial septum and left atrium with pericardial effusion. In a 27 year old man who presented with progressive dyspnea.

4. Metastatic cardiac tumors

Metastatic tumors are 20 to 40 times more common than primary malignant ones with prevalence of 6% in post-mortem autopsies in malignant diseases (6).

4.1 Malignant melanoma

For the first time the term "melanotic heart" was introduced by William Norris in 1820 (7). However, many cases of malignant melanoma have been described in scientific literature.

Malignant melanoma frequently (50-71%) metastasizes to the heart (19). It seems to have the highest rate of metastases to heart. When a patient presents with cardiac metastases of melanoma, the disease has already spread throughout the body and is rarely curable (20). Single metastasis is rare. Metastases could be found in right side or left side; however, bilateral metastasis is frequently seen (21). The way of tumor spread toward heart is mostly hematogenous as seen in lymphoma and leukemia.

Previously, histologic diagnosis of malignant melanoma was made postmortem; however, with early detection of metastases due to availability of new imaging modalities, definite antemortem diagnosis and pathologic examination is frequently possible. Tissue specimen can be obtained by echocardiography guided transvenous biopsy or by resection of mass (22).

The symptoms are nonspecific such as chronic pericarditis, congestive heart failure, pericardial effusion, tamponade, conduction disturbances or defects, arrhythmias such as ventricular or supraventricular heart rhythm disturbances (23,24), syncope, embolism events such as transient ischemic attack and hemodynamic changes secondary to valve dysfunction.

Malignant melanoma has the highest rate of metastases to heart; however, due to improvement in treatment for this disease, longer survival than previous is now possible (25) and with newer imaging modalities early detection of metastases is possible and the physician should be alert of the risk of metastases. Transesophageal echocardiography has higher sensitivity than transthoracic echocardiography and cardiac magnetic resonance imaging with its ability to define the mediastinal involvement could also be used. According to tumor characteristics, its burden, location and size, palliative surgery or complete resection or adjuvant systemic therapy is recommended.

5. Summary

Echocardiography both transthoracic echocardiography (TTE), transesophageal echocardiography (TEE), is the commonly available noninvasive method for the diagnosis of cardiac masses. Tumor size, location and texture, and its extension to adjacent organs, its attachment to cardiac structures, presence or absence of pericardial effusion, interference with valve function, any obstruction and tumor mobility could be evaluated by echocardiography. In patients with poor echo window, TEE gives superior results, however, in some patients for better evaluation of cardiac tumor and its extension, other imaging modalities such as MRI is needed. Extra cardiac structures could be visualized better in TTE then TEE which is important for surgeons for choosing the most suitable plan for surgery(7).

6. Acknowledgement

Special thanks to doctor Hyderi for his valuable comments.

7. References

[1] Reynen K. Frequency of primary tumors of the heart. Am J Cardiol 1996;77: 107.
[2] Reynen K. Cardiac myxomas. N Engl J Med 1995; 333: 1610–1617.

[3] Libby P, Bonow R, Mann DL, Zipes DP. Braunwald's Heart Disease: A Textbook of Cardiovascular Medicine, 8th edition

[4] Roberts WC, Glancy DL, DeVita VT. Heart in malignant lymphoma. A study of 196 autopsy cases. Am J Cardiol 1968;22: 85–107

[5] Silverman J, Olwin JS, Graettinger JS. Cardiac myxomas with systemic embolization review of the literature and report of a case. Circulation 1962; 26: 99–10

[6] Hoffmann U, Globits S, Frank H, Cardiac and paracardiac masses Current opinion on diagnostic evaluation by magnetic resonance imaging . Eur Heart J (1998) 19, 553–563.

[7] McAllister Jr HA, Fenoglio Jr JJ. Tumors of the cardiovascular system. Atlas of tumor pathology, 2nd series. Fascicle 15 Washington, D. C. Armed Forces Institute of Pathology, 1978:1–20.

[8] Otto CM. The Practice of Clinical Echocardiography. 3rd edition. 2008, pp. 1108-1131.

[9] Edwards FH, Hale D, Cohen A, et al: Primary cardiac valve tumors. Ann Thoracic Surg 1991; 52:1127-31.

[10] Klarich KW, Enriquez Sarano M, Gura GM, Edwards WD, Tajik AJ, Seward JB. Papillary fibroelastoma:Echocardiographic Characteristics for diagnosis and pathologic correlation Am Coll Cardiol 1997;30:784-790.

[11] Mugge A, Daniel WG, Haverich A, et al: Diagnosis of non-infective cardiac mss lesions by two-dimensional echocardiography. Comparison of the transthoracic and transesophageal approaches. Circulation 1991; 83:70-78.

[12] Winkler M, Higgins CB: Suspected intracardiac masses: Evaluation with MR imaging. Radiol 1987; 165:117-122.

[13] Sun JP, Ashe CR, Yang XS, Cheng GG, Scalia GM, Massed AG, Griffin BP, Ratlift NB, Stewart WJ, Thomas JD. Clinical and echocardiographic characteristics of papillary fibroelastoma : a retrospective and prospective study in 162 patients. Circulation 2001;103:2687-93.

[14] Lichtenstein HL, Lee JC, Stewart S. Papillary tumor of the heart:incidental finding at surgery. Hum pathol 1979;10:473-5.

[15] Mc Alister HA, Fenoglio JJ. Tumors of the cardiovascular system. In: Atrak of tumor pathology second series fascicle 15. Washington DC Armed Forces Institute of pathology, 1978; 20-25.

[16] Roberts WC, Papillary Fibroelastoma of the heart. Am J Cardiol 1997; 80:973-975.

[17] Hicks KA, Kovach JA, Frishberg DP, Wiley TM, Gurezak PB, Vernalis MN. Echocardiographic evaluation of papillary fibroelastoma: a case report and review of the literature. Am J Soc Echocardiogr 1996;9:353-60

[18] Almagro UA, Perry LS, Choi H, Pinator K. Papillary fibroelastoma of the heart. Report of six cases. Arch Pathol Lab Med. 1982;106:318-321

[19] latt EC, Heiz DR, Cardiac Metastases. Cancer 1990;65:1456-9

[20] Chen RH, Gaos CM, Frazier OH. Complete resection of a right atrial intracavitary metastatic melanoma. Annals thoracic surgery 1996;61:1255-7

[21] Reynen K, Köckeritz U, Strasser R. H. Metastases to the heart Annals of Oncology 2004;15:375–381.

[22] Rubin DC, Ziskind AA, Hawke MW, Plotnick GD. Transesophageal echocardiographically guided percutaneous biopsy of a right atrial mass. Am Heart J 1994;127:935-6.

[23] Lin TK, Stech JM, Eckert WG, Liu JJ et al. Pericardial angiosarcomata simulating pericardial effusion by echography. Chest 1978; 73: 881–3.

[24] Coghlan JG, Paul VE, Mitchell AG. Cardiac involvement by lymphoma. Diagnostic difficulties. Eur Heart J 1989; 10:765–8

[25] Samiei N, Moshkani Farahani M, Sadeghipour A, Mozaffari K, Maleki M. Intracardiac metastasis of malignant melanoma. European Journal of Echocardiography (2008) 9, 393–394.

10

Echocardiography in Kawasaki Disease

Deane Yim, David Burgner and Michael Cheung
*Department of Cardiology, Royal Children's Hospital
and Murdoch Childrens Research Institute,
Heart Research Group, Melbourne
Australia*

1. Introduction

Kawasaki disease is an acute childhood systemic vasculitis characterised by a number of clinical features, with a predilection for damage to the coronary arteries. It predominantly affects children between the ages of 6 months to 4 years, although cases at either extreme of childhood are well described and are recognised to be associated with a greater risk of delayed diagnosis and treatment (Harnden et al., 2009; Pannaraj et al., 2004). There is a male predominance with a male to female ratio of 1.6 to 1. Despite important research progress since its first description in 1967 (Kawasaki, 1967), the aetiology remains unknown and there is no diagnostic test. The timely use of intravenous immunoglobulin has reduced the incidence of coronary artery lesions from 25% to 2-4% (Newburger et al., 2004). Transthoracic echocardiography is recommended in suspected cases of KD, however a normal study does not exclude the diagnosis.

2. Incidence

Kawasaki disease is the most common cause of paediatric acquired heart disease (Taubert et al., 1991). The incidence has been rising in both developed (Japan, Korea and United Kingdom) and rapidly industrialising countries such as India, which may reflect both a genuine increase and increased recognition (Krishnakumar & Mathews, 2006). The highest annual incidence is reported in Japan (218 per 100000 children <5 years of age) and Korea (113 per 100000 <5 years) (Nakamura et al., 2010; Park et al., 2011). The incidence is lower in Australia (3.7 per 100000 <5 years) but this data is 15 years old (Royle et al., 1998); given the rising incidence in other countries these rates may be an underestimate of true disease burden. Current epidemiological research is in progress in Western Australia, and these data will provide an updated incidence for Australia children.

3. Aetiology

The high incidence of Kawasaki disease in Asian populations and increased risk in families and siblings suggests a genetic predisposition (Fujita et al., 1989; Uehara et al., 2003). Seasonal patterns are well recognised, with peaks in winter and spring in Australia, the United States and Europe and spring to summer peaks in Korea and China (Burgner &

Harnden, 2005). The epidemiology of Kawasaki disease, clustering of cases, community outbreaks and epidemics in the 1980s, support the hypothesis that an unknown infectious agent (or agents) triggers an abnormal inflammatory response in genetically susceptible individuals. Both conventional antigens and bacterial superantigens have been implicated as causative triggers in Kawasaki disease, however the triggering pathogen(s) remain unknown.

4. Pathogenesis

Initially, activated inflammatory cells, particularly monocytes, macrophages, T-cells, and subsequently platelets, adhere to the endothelial cells that line medium-size elastic arteries. Other mediators contribute to destruction of the extra-cellular matrix, leading to vessel dilatation, and subsequent smooth muscle proliferation in the media contributes to later pathology. There is destruction of the intimal layer of the affected artery with inflammatory infiltrate during the acute phase, and histologic findings of myocarditis and fibrosis are found in virtually all cases with Kawasaki disease (Yutani et al., 1981).

5. Clinical assessment

The typical presentation is of an irritable child who has an unremitting high fever (often >39°C) for 5 or more days, and some or all classical diagnostic of the clinical features (Table 1). The diagnosis can also be made by experienced clinicians on the fourth day of fever if classical diagnostic criteria are met.[1] In most children the clinical features appear sequentially. Specific features for KD include perineal desquamation and erythema or crusting around the Bacille Calmette Guerin (BCG) inoculation site. Other extracardiac features such as respiratory or gastrointestinal symptoms occur frequently and make the diagnosis difficult.

The diagnosis requires the presence of fever for at least 5 days, and at least four of the following five criteria:

-   Polymorphous rash
-   Oral mucous membrane involvement, including red fissured lips, strawberry tongue or injected pharynx
-   Bilateral non-exudative conjunctivitis
-   Changes with extremities including erythema or oedema of palms and soles, or periungal desquamation as a late sign in the subacute phase (~2 or more weeks after illness onset)
-   Cervical lymphadenopathy, defined as a unilateral lymph node of ≥1.5cm

---

Table 1. The diagnostic criteria for Kawasaki disease (Newburger et al. 2004)

Incomplete KD should be considered in children who have an unexplained prolonged febrile illness and have not met diagnostic criteria (Newburger et al., 2004). This occurs more commonly in children less than 6 months or greater than 5 years of age, with the younger age group more likely to present with fewer clinical features and also a higher incidence of coronary artery abnormalities (Genizi et al., 2003).

Kawasaki disease shock syndrome has been recently described and is characterised by hypotension and haemodynamic instability, often requiring intensive care. (Dominguez et al., 2008; Yim et al., 2010) These patients may be at increased risk of delayed diagnosis and treatment, refractory disease and more severe coronary artery involvement (Kanegaye et al., 2009).

6. Echocardiography in Kawasaki disease

Transthoracic echocardiography is highly sensitive and specific for the diagnosis of coronary artery involvement and should be performed in confirmed or suspected cases of Kawasaki disease at the time of diagnosis. It is important to ensure that the timing or results of the echocardiogram do not delay initial treatment of Kawasaki disease, and that the diagnosis is made predominantly on clinical findings. On the other hand, if full criteria are not met and coronary artery abnormalities are present on echocardiography, then the child has incomplete features of Kawasaki disease and treatment with high dose intravenous immunoglobulin should be considered. The American Heart Association consensus guidelines provide a schema for the incorporation of echocardiography into the diagnostic process in children with possible incomplete Kawasaki disease (Newburger et al., 2004).

7. Principles of echocardiographic assessment

7.1 Optimisation of imaging modalities

The primary aim of echocardiography is to identify coronary artery involvement, pericarditis and/or myocarditis. As always, optimising machine settings, using the highest possible frequency transducer and reducing two-dimensional gain and compression can achieve better image quality and resolution. B-mode cine loops and still frame images are necessary to assess coronary artery calibre, along with colour Doppler imaging set at a low Nyquist limit for evaluating normal coronary artery diastolic flow. Sedation may be necessary in children who are too irritable to tolerate a detailed study; our preference is to use 50-100mg/kg of chloral hydrate (max 1g) given orally with heart rate and peripheral oxygen saturation monitoring.

7.2 Coronary artery assessment

Coronary arteries should be assessed in multiple imaging planes before a decision is reached about the presence or absence of coronary artery abnormalities. The parasternal short axis view with or without a clockwise rotation of the transducer allows for imaging of the left coronary artery origin, left anterior descending artery and left circumflex artery, as well as the right coronary artery origin and proximal course. Parasternal long axis views with sweeps between the aorta and pulmonary artery will delineate the left main coronary artery, left anterior descending and circumflex arteries. Subcostal views are helpful for assessing the left circumflex artery and the mid-course of the right coronary artery. Apical four chamber views will show the length of the left circumflex artery and distal right coronary artery in the left and right atrioventricular grooves respectively. Coronary artery measurements should be taken from the inner edge to inner edge of the vessel wall and should not be measured at the level of normal branching.

8. Cardiovascular involvement

8.1 Coronary artery involvement

The main features of coronary artery involvement are dilatation, aneurysm formation, lack of tapering of the distal coronary vessel and perivascular brightness. Aneurysms may be fusiform (spindle-shaped, gradual tapering from normal to dilated segment), saccular (spherical, acute transition from normal to dilated segment), ectatic (uniformly dilated long segment) or segmented (multiple dilatations joined by normal or stenotic areas) (Figure 1). The common sites of coronary involvement (from highest to lowest frequency) include the proximal left anterior descending artery (Figure 2), proximal right coronary artery (Figure 3 & 4), left main coronary artery (Figure 5), left circumflex branch (Figure 5), distal right coronary artery (Figure 6) and the junction of the right and posterior descending coronary artery. Takahashi et al reported that aneurysms were more likely to resolve if they were fusiform in nature and if the child was female and/or less than a year of age. Distal coronary artery aneurysms tended to regress more rapidly than aneurysms located in proximal coronary vessels (Takahashi et al., 1987).

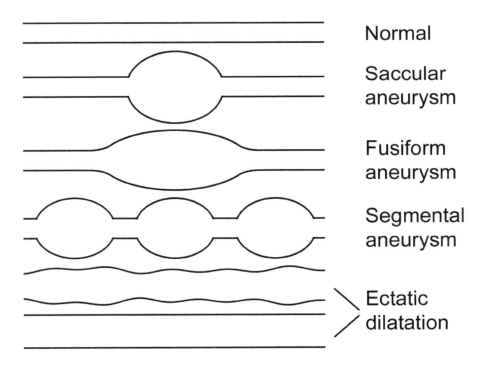

Fig. 1. Illustrative example of coronary artery abnormalities.

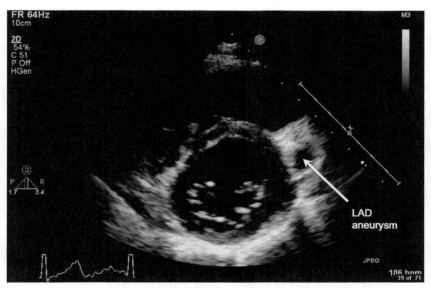

Fig. 2. Parasternal short axis echocardiographic image at the level of the mitral valve leaflets demonstrating an aneurysm of the left anterior descending artery.

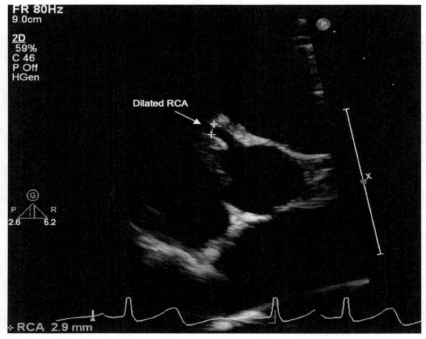

Fig. 3. Parasternal short axis echocardiographic image showing a uniformly dilated proximal right coronary artery (RCA).

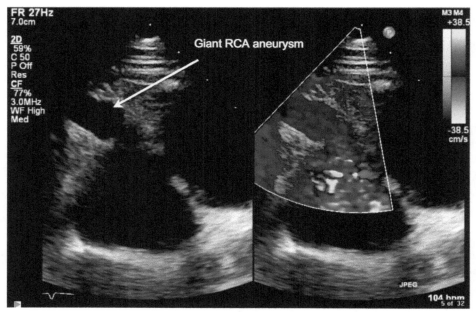

Fig. 4. Parasternal short axis image showing a giant aneurysm of the right coronary artery (RCA).

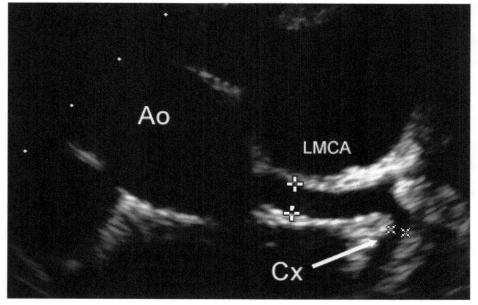

Fig. 5. Parasternal short axis view showing a uniformly dilated left main coronary artery (LMCA, 4.7mm) and dilated circumflex artery (Cx, 3.4mm). Ao = aorta

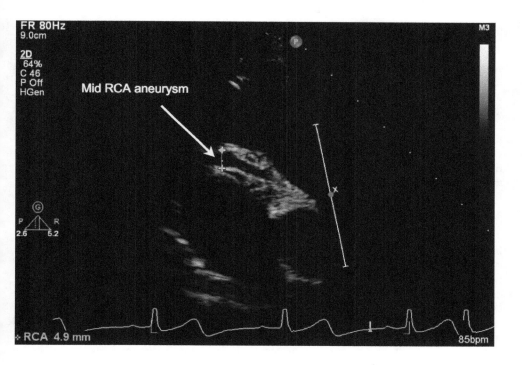

Fig. 6. Off-axis parasternal short axis view demonstrating a fusiform aneurysm of the mid to distal right coronary artery (RCA) aneurysm

8.2 Myo-pericarditis

Virtually all patients with Kawasaki disease develop myocarditis to varying degrees during the acute phase, and over half of these patients develop acute transient left ventricular dysfunction (Ajami et al., 2010). Systolic left ventricular function should be routinely assessed. Regional wall motion abnormalities may occur if there is significant coronary artery involvement. Pericarditis may be reflected by the presence of a pericardial effusion.

8.3 Valvar involvement

Myocardial inflammation may also involve valve tissue and lead to mitral, tricuspid or aortic regurgitation that is usually mild in nature. If severe mitral regurgitation is present, papillary muscle dysfunction and myocardial ischaemia should be assessed (Akagi et al., 1990). Mild aortic regurgitation is seen to persist in approximately 4% of patients with serial follow-up (Ravekes et al., 2001). Aortic root dilatation may occur as part of the overall vasculitis but is usually mild.

9. Timing of echocardiography

The consensus statement from the American Heart Association recommends performing echocardiography at diagnosis, 2 weeks and repeating at 6-8 weeks after the onset of illness for uncomplicated cases. In some centres the 2 week echocardiogram is not routinely performed. The imaging at diagnosis should provide a baseline study for serial follow-up of left ventricular function, coronary arterial involvement, valvar regurgitation, myocarditis and/or a pericardial effusion. The presence of any cardiac involvement warrants closer follow-up. In particular, coronary aneurysms > 5mm in size require close monitoring because of an elevated risk of developing stenotic lesions within the vessel (Mueller, 2009). By 6-8 weeks, transient cardiac involvement is likely to have resolved, or if coronary artery dilation and/or aneurysms are present, the maximum diameter is usually reached by this time.

10. Definitions of coronary artery involvement

A number of definitions have been proposed to describe and quantitate coronary artery involvement. The Japanese Ministry of Health classification was first published in 1984. Aneurysms are considered to be small if their internal diameter is <5mm, medium if between 5-8mm, or giant if the internal diameter of the aneurysm is >8mm (Figure 5). These criteria are widely used and define absolute values for coronary artery dimensions and therefore do not account for differences in patient size or the usual caliber of different coronary artery branches. The American Heart Association AHA guidelines were published in 2004 and define coronary artery dimensions with respect to body surface area, which requires both weight and height measurements. These define a coronary artery as dilated if the intra-luminal diameter has a z-score of ≥ 2.5mm. Manlhiot et al. recently proposed a revision of this classification to account for differences in body size and caliber of coronary artery branches, and report that coronary artery abnormalities are small if the z-score is ≥ 2.5 to <5, large if the z-score is ≥ 5 to < 10, and giant if the z-score is ≥ 10 (Manlhiot et al., 2010). This method is however prone to significant variation in the calculated z-score with minor variation in measurement of coronary size. It is therefore too early to determine whether this classification will be widely employed.

11. Further imaging modalities

As the difficulty of coronary artery imaging increases with age, further imaging options may be necessary. Even in experienced hands, echocardiography also has its limitations in detecting stenosis and thrombosis. The efficacy of other non-invasive imaging modalities such as magnetic resonance imaging and multi-detector computed tomography has been increasingly evaluated for coronary artery assessment in Kawasaki disease (Figure 7).

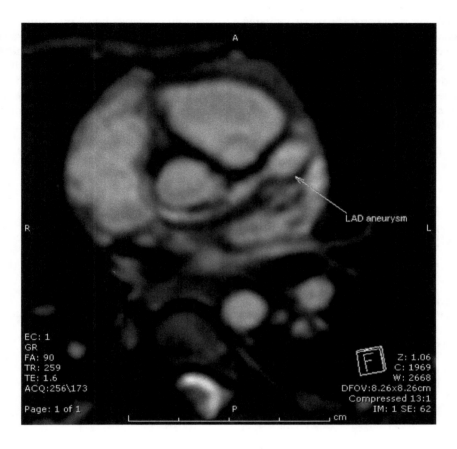

Fig. 7. Magnetic resonance image using T2 weighted truFISP sequence demonstrating a dilated left anterior descending (LAD) artery with a distal fusiform aneurysm.

12. Functional assessment

Cardiac stress testing may be used to identify reversible ischaemia and regional wall motion abnormalities during increased demand. Coronary perfusion abnormalities can be further assessed with exercise echocardiography, pharmacologic (dobutamine, dipyridamole or adenosine) stress echocardiography and exercise myocardial perfusion scans. The stress modality employed depends on the age of the child and local expertise, although practically speaking, pharmacologic stress echocardiography or exercise myocardial perfusion scans are the preferred techniques in the paediatric age group. If abnormalities of coronary segmental perfusion are found, the results may assist decision-making for further management.

13. Cardiac catheterisation

Cardiac catheterisation with selective coronary angiography is considered the gold standard for delineation of coronary artery anatomy, and if required interventional procedures such as balloon angioplasty, stent placement or percutaneous transluminal coronary revascularisation may be performed in the same setting. Cardiac catheterisation is generally not recommended for patients with mild coronary artery involvement, however it can provide useful detailed information and help with risk stratification of patients who have complex coronary artery lesions (Figure 8 & 9). Coronary angiography in this instance is recommended 6-12 months after the onset of Kawasaki disease, or sooner as clinically indicated.

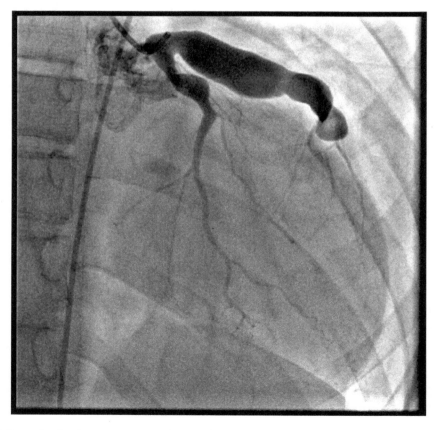

Fig. 8. Lateral selective coronary angiogram demonstrating a significantly dilated left anterior descending (LAD) artery and proximal circumflex (Cx) artery.

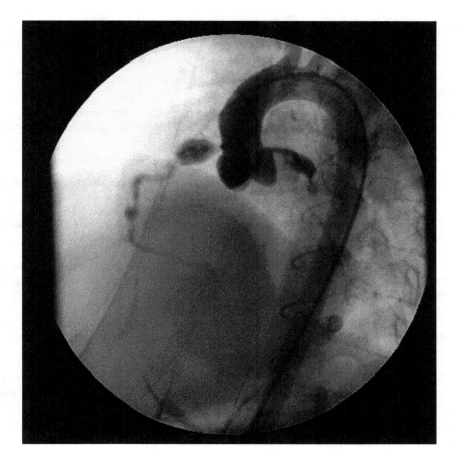

Fig. 9. Lateral angiographic plane with injection of contrast in the ascending aorta via a pigtail catheter, showing large saccular aneurysms in both the proximal right and left coronary arteries. (Image courtesy of Professor Mike South, Royal Children's Hopsital, Melbourne)

14. Natural history

The percentage of patients developing coronary aneurysms is reduced with timely administration of intravenous immunoglobulin. Nearly 50% of those coronary artery aneurysms will show angiographic regression within 1 to 2 years following the illness, with smaller lesions having a greater chance of resolution (Newburger et al., 2004). The size of the aneurysm is a major predictor for the development of myocardial infarction (Yeu et al., 2008). As aneurysms remodel with time, however, the risk of coronary artery stenosis increases.

There is evidence that Kawasaki disease in childhood may increase the risk of cardiovascular disease in adulthood. Patients with coronary artery aneurysms have an increase in carotid artery intima-media thickness, and increased systemic arterial stiffness with higher pulse wave velocities (Cheung et al., 2007; Ooyanagi et al., 2004; Suzuki et al., 1996). Furthermore there are data demonstrating abnormal vascular endothelial function and lipid profiles in patients. The exact level of increased risk is uncertain.

15. Follow-up recommendations

Patients with Kawasaki disease should be followed up based on risk stratification according to the severity of coronary artery involvement in consultation with a paediatric cardiologist familiar with managing the condition.

- **Kawasaki disease is a common childhood systemic vasculitis characterized by specific clinical features and persistent fever for at least 5 days.**

- **Transthoracic echocardiography is recommended in suspected cases of Kawasaki disease, however a normal study does not exclude the diagnosis.**

- **Treatment with high dose intravenous immunoglobulin should be initiated based on the clinical presentation, and should not be delayed by the timing of echocardiography.**

- **The aims of echocardiography are to identify coronary artery dilatation and aneurysms, valvar regurgitation, myocarditis with ventricular dysfunction and pericarditis with effusion.**

- **Echocardiography should be performed at diagnosis, and approximately 6-8 weeks after the onset of illness, with more frequent assessments required if cardiac involvement is present.**

Table 2. Kawasaki disease - Summary points

16. Conclusion

In summary, Kawasaki disease is an important and common systemic vasculitis of childhood, and the advent of intravenous immunoglobulin has significantly reduced, but not removed the risk of abnormal coronary artery development in affected individuals. There have been significant advances in our overall understanding of the condition, although the aetiology remains uncertain. Of concern is the emerging evidence that KD is a risk factor for adult coronary artery disease. Further research into pathogenesis and long term outcomes are required.

17. Acknowledgements

We would like to thank Professor Mike South for his contribution of catheterisation images, and Dr Adam Doyle for the coronary artery illustration.

18. References

Ajami, G, Borzouee, M, Ammozgar, H, Ashnaee, F & Kashef, S et al. (2010) Evaluation of myocardial function using the Tei index in patients with Kawasaki disease. *Cardiol Young.* Feb;20(1):44-8

Akagi, T, Kato, H, Inoue, O et al. (1990) Valvular heart disease in Kawasaki syndrome: incidence and natural history. *Am Heart J,* 120:366-72.

Burgner, D & Harnden, A. (2005) Kawasaki disease: what is the epidemiology telling us about the etiology? *Int J Infect Dis,* 9:185-194

Cheung, Y, Wong, S, Ho, M. (2007) Relationship between carotid intima-media thickness and arterial stiffness in children after Kawasaki disease. *Arch Dis Child,* Jan;92(1):43-7

Harnden, A, Takahashi, M &Burgner, D. (2009) Kawasaki disease. *BMJ.* May 5;338:b1514

Dominguez, S, Friedman, K, Seewald, R, Anderson, M & Willis, L et al. (2008) Kawasaki disease in a pediatric intensive care unit: a case-control study. *Pediatrics.* Oct;122(4):e786-90

Duerinckx, A, Troutman B, Allada, V, Kim, D. Coronary MR angiography in Kawasaki disease. (1997) *Am J Roentgenol.* Jan;168(1):114-6

Fujita, Y, Nakamura, Y, Sakata, K, Hara, N & Kobayashi, M et al. (1989) Kawasaki disease in families. *Pediatrics.* Oct;84(4):666-9

Genizi, J, Miron, D, Spiegel, R, Fink, D & Horowitz, Y. (2003) Kawasaki disease in very young infants: high prevalence of atypical presentation and coronary arteritis. *Clin Pediatr (Phila).* Apr;42(3):263-7

Kanegaye, J, Wilder, M, Molkara, D, Frazer, J & Pancheri, J et al. (2009) Recognition of a Kawasaki disease shock syndrome. *Pediatrics.* May;123(5):e783-9

Kawasaki, T. (1967) Acute febrile mucocutaneous syndrome with lymphoid involvement with specific desquamation of the fingers and toes in children. *Arerugi.* Mar;16(3):178-222

Krishnakumar, P & Mathews, L. (2006) Kawasaki disease is not rare in India. *Indian J Pediatr.* Jun;73(6):544-5

Manlhiot, C, Millar, K, Golding, F & McCrindle, B. (2010) Improved classification of coronary artery abnormalities based only on coronary artery z-scores after Kawasaki disease. . *Pediatr Cardiol.* Feb;31(2):242-9. Epub 2009 Dec 19

Mueller, F, Knirsch, W, Harpes, P, Pretre, R & Valsangiacomo, E et al. (2009) Long-term follow-up of acute changes in coronary artery diameter caused by Kawasaki disease: risk factors for development of stenotic lesions. *Clin Res Cardiol.* Aug;98(8):501-7.

Nakamura, Y, Yashiro, M, Uehara, R, Sadakane, A & Chihara, I et al. Epidemiologic features of Kawasaki disease in Japan: results of the 2007-2008 nationwide survey. *J Epidemiol.* 20(4):302-7

Newburger, J, Takahashi, M, Gerber, M, Gerwitz, M & Tani, L et al. (2004) Diagnosis, treatment, and long-term management of Kawasaki disease: a statement for health professionals from the Committee on Rheumatic Fever, Endocarditis and Kawasaki Disease, Council on Cardiovascular Disease in the Young, American Heart Association. *Circulation.* Oct 26;110(17):2747-71

Ooyanagi, R, Fuse, S, Tomita, H, Takamuro, M & Horita, N et al. (2004) Pulse wave velocity and ankle brachial index in patients with Kawasaki disease. *Pediatr Int.* Aug;46(4):398-402

Pannaraj, P, Turner, C, Bastian, J & Burns, J. (2004) Failure to diagnose Kawasaki disease at the extremes of the pediatric age range. *Pediatr Infect Dis J.* Aug;23(8):789

Park, Y, Han, J, Hong, Y, Ma, J & Cha, S et al. (2011) Epidemiological features of Kawasaki disease in Korea, 2006-2008. *Pediatr Int.* Feb;53(1):36-9

Ravekes, W, Colan, S, Gauvreau, K, Baker, A & Sundel, R et al. (2001) Aortic root dilation in Kawasaki disease. *Am J Cardiol.* 87: 919–922

Royle, J, Williams, K, Elliott, E, Sholler, G & Nolan, T et al. (1998) Kawasaki disease in Australia, 1993-95. *Arch Dis Child.* Jan;78(1):33-39

Suzuki, A, Yamagishi, M, Kimura, K, Sugiyama, H & Arakaki, Y et al. (1996) Functional behavior and morphology of the coronary artery wall in patients with Kawasaki disease assessed by intravascular ultrasound. *J Am Coll Cardiol.* Feb;27(2):291-6

Takahashi, M, Mason, W & Lewis, A. (1987) Regression of coronary artery aneurysms in patients with Kawasaki syndrome. *Circulation.* Feb;75(2):387-94

Taubert, K, Rowley, A & Shulman, S. (1991) Nationwide survey of Kawasaki disease and acute rheumatic fever. *J Pediatr.* 119: 279–282

Uehara, R, Yashiro, M, Nakamura, Y & Yanagawa, H. (2003) Kawasaki disease in parents and children. *Acta Paediatr.* Jun;92(6):694-7

Yeu, B, Menahem, S, Goldstein, J. (2008) Giant coronary artery aneurysms in Kawasaki disease – the need for coronary artery bypass. *Heart Lung Circ.* Oct;17(5):404-6

Yim, D, Ramsay, J, Kothari, D & Burgner, D et al. (2010) Coronary artery dilatation in toxic shock-like syndrome: the Kawasaki disease shock syndrome. *Pediatr Cardiol* Nov;31(8):1232-5

Yutani, C, Go, S, Kamiya, T, Hirose, O & Misawa, H. (1981) Cardiac biopsy of Kawasaki disease. *Arch Pathol Lab Med.* Sep;105(9):470-3

Permissions

The contributors of this book come from diverse backgrounds, making this book a truly international effort. This book will bring forth new frontiers with its revolutionizing research information and detailed analysis of the nascent developments around the world.

We would like to thank Prof.Asoc.Gani Bajraktari, MD, MSc, PhD, FESC, FACC, for lending his expertise to make the book truly unique. He has played a crucial role in the development of this book. Without his invaluable contribution this book wouldn't have been possible. He has made vital efforts to compile up to date information on the varied aspects of this subject to make this book a valuable addition to the collection of many professionals and students.

This book was conceptualized with the vision of imparting up-to-date information and advanced data in this field. To ensure the same, a matchless editorial board was set up. Every individual on the board went through rigorous rounds of assessment to prove their worth. After which they invested a large part of their time researching and compiling the most relevant data for our readers. Conferences and sessions were held from time to time between the editorial board and the contributing authors to present the data in the most comprehensible form. The editorial team has worked tirelessly to provide valuable and valid information to help people across the globe.

Every chapter published in this book has been scrutinized by our experts. Their significance has been extensively debated. The topics covered herein carry significant findings which will fuel the growth of the discipline. They may even be implemented as practical applications or may be referred to as a beginning point for another development. Chapters in this book were first published by InTech; hereby published with permission under the Creative Commons Attribution License or equivalent.

The editorial board has been involved in producing this book since its inception. They have spent rigorous hours researching and exploring the diverse topics which have resulted in the successful publishing of this book. They have passed on their knowledge of decades through this book. To expedite this challenging task, the publisher supported the team at every step. A small team of assistant editors was also appointed to further simplify the editing procedure and attain best results for the readers.

Our editorial team has been hand-picked from every corner of the world. Their multi-ethnicity adds dynamic inputs to the discussions which result in innovative outcomes. These outcomes are then further discussed with the researchers and contributors who give their valuable feedback and opinion regarding the same. The feedback is then collaborated with the researches and they are edited in a comprehensive manner to aid the understanding of the subject.

Apart from the editorial board, the designing team has also invested a significant amount of their time in understanding the subject and creating the most relevant covers. They scrutinized every image to scout for the most suitable representation of the subject and create an appropriate cover for the book.

The publishing team has been involved in this book since its early stages. They were actively engaged in every process, be it collecting the data, connecting with the contributors or procuring relevant information. The team has been an ardent support to the editorial, designing and production team. Their endless efforts to recruit the best for this project, has resulted in the accomplishment of this book. They are a veteran in the field of academics and their pool of knowledge is as vast as their experience in printing. Their expertise and guidance has proved useful at every step. Their uncompromising quality standards have made this book an exceptional effort. Their encouragement from time to time has been an inspiration for everyone.

The publisher and the editorial board hope that this book will prove to be a valuable piece of knowledge for researchers, students, practitioners and scholars across the globe.

List of Contributors

Gani Bajraktari
Service of Cardiology, University Clinical Centre of Kosova, Prishtina, Republic of Kosovo

Gheorghe Cerin, Bogdan Adrian Popa and Marco Diena
The Cardioteam Foundation / San Gaudenzio Clinic, Novara, Italy

Alistair Royse
Department of Surgery, The Royal Melbourne Hospital, Australia

Colin Royse
Pharmacology, The University of Melbourne, The Royal Melbourne Hospital, Australia

Ryotaro Wake, Junichi Yoshikawa and Minoru Yoshiyama
Osaka City University Graduate School of Medicine, Japan

Dawod Sharif and Uri Rosenschein
Cardiology Department, Bnai Zion Medical Center, Haifa, Israel
Technion, Israel Institute of Technology, Haifa, Israel

Amal Sharif-Rasslan
Technion, Israel Institute of Technology, Haifa, Israel
Mathematics Departmant, The Academic Arab College, Haifa, Israel

Fadi N. Salloum and Rakesh C. Kukreja
Virginia Commonwealth University, Medical Center Richmond, Virginia, USA

Toru Maruyama
Institute of Health Science, Japan

Yousuke Kokawa, Hisataka Nakamura, Mitsuhiro Fukata, Shioto Yasuda, Keita Odashiro and Koichi Akashi
Department of Medicine, Kyushu University, Fukuoka, Japan

Yi-Chia Wang and Chi-Hsiang Huang
National Taiwan University Hospital, Taiwan, R.O.C.

Maryam Moshkani Farahani
Department of Echocardiography, Faculty of Medicine, Baqiyatallah University of Medical Sciences, Molla Sadra Avenue, Tehran, Iran

Deane Yim, David Burgner and Michael Cheung
Department of Cardiology, Royal Children's Hospital and Murdoch Childrens Research Institute, Heart Research Group, Melbourne, Australia